The 3:00 PM S

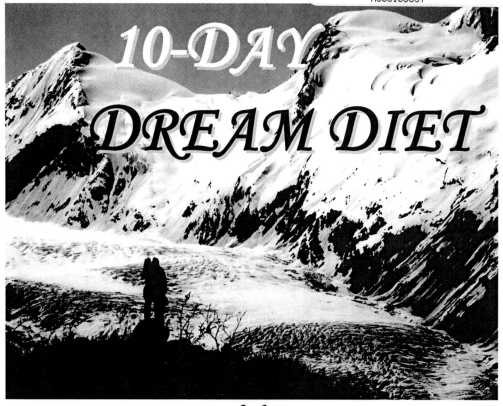

10-DAY

DREAM DIET

Including

Lifestyle Secrets and Inspirations from Alaska to the World

Debra Anne Ross Lawrence

With Musings by

David Allen Lawrence

GlacierDog Publishing

A Division of GlacierDog Intergalactica

Anchorage, Alaska

THE 3:00 PM SECRET 10-DAY DREAM DIET

Lifestyle Secrets and Inspirations from Alaska to the World

Copyright 2010 Debra Anne Ross Lawrence
David Allen Lawrence (Contributing Author)

ISBN 978-0-9797459-1-1
ISBN 0-9797459-1-8

Library of Congress Control Number: 2009911803

Notice to the Reader

The author and publisher have done their best to present accurate and up-to-date information in this book, but cannot guarantee that the information is correct or will suit your particular situation. If you do anything recommended in this book without the supervision of a licensed medical doctor or other appropriate professional advisor, you do so at your own risk. The author and publisher present this information for educational purposes only and do not attempt to prescribe any medical treatment. If you require expert assistance, you should obtain this assistance from a qualified professional.

TABLE OF CONTENTS

Acknowledgements

I would first like to thank my wonderful husband and contributing author, David Lawrence, for writing the insightful, informative, and amusing Male Musings, and for providing ideas and editing.

This book also benefited greatly from the creativity and wisdom of my amazing mother, Maggie Ross. I appreciate her many suggestions and edits.

I would like to express deep appreciation to my friend, Connie, who I got to know as she tested the *Dream Diet* and provided her thoughts and insights.

Many thanks to Noah Joraanstad, our favorite Alaska pilot, for his expert photography of Portage Glacier that graces the cover of the book.

I truly appreciate Robert German's expertise in providing the final formatting of the book's cover.

I would like to thank the readers of *The 3:00 PM Secret: Live Slim and Strong Live Your Dreams.* I truly appreciate their many thoughtful questions and comments. Appendix 4 of this book addresses Frequently Asked Questions from those who contacted me through www.glacierdog.com or spoke to me in person.

The concept of presenting *The 3:00 PM Secret* lifestyle in a simple 10-day formula as a stand-alone book with an emphasis on how to discover and create your dream life evolved from conversations with David Lawrence, Maggie Ross, my sister Jan Ross, my good friend Kathy Williams, and readers of *The 3:00 PM Secret.* Many thanks to each of you.

Dare to Dream

Adopt the 3:00 PM SECRET Lifestyle

Follow the Ten Nutrition Tips

Discover Your Dreams

Do the Ten-Minute Workout

Sleep Adequately

Dare to Live Your Dreams!

Is This Book For You?

Have you tried and failed at countless weight-loss plans and lost hope you will ever master your weight? Are you missing out on the life you had hoped for and have you just about given up on your dreams? Do you feel as if your body is out of control and is standing between you and your dreams? If this sounds familiar, I wrote *The 10-Day Dream Diet* especially for you.

The 10-Day Dream Diet shows you how to achieve your dream body and just how simple it is to control your weight. It provides a simple, straightforward *weight-loss* formula that includes following *The 3:00 PM Secret* lifestyle, easy daily menus, simple exercises you can do at home in minutes, and nutrition and lifestyle wisdom from *Alaska to the World*. Together these will give you quick and *sustainable* weight loss. You will find that obtaining and maintaining your dream body is surprisingly easy.

The 10-Day Dream Diet also coaches you toward the discovery of your dream life using revealing *Dream* questions. After following *The 10-Day Dream Diet* and working through your *Dream* questions for a 10-day period, you will have new hope and motivation. You will realize that the fit body and wonderful life you desire are within reach!

Note to the Reader…

In the mid-1990's I began researching and developing *The 3:00 PM Secret* lifestyle in response to a prolonged, serious illness. I was determined to regain my strength and health and, at the same time, figure out what I truly wanted to do with the rest of my life. Using my scientific training and resources, I gathered the latest, most comprehensive information on health, wellness, and longevity available. In 2007 *The 3:00 PM Secret: Live Slim and Strong Live Your Dreams* was published. In that book I describe the philosophy and practical steps that made me slim, strong, and healthy. I explain the *Secret*; provide key information on nutrition, sleep, aging, and exercise; and explain how to gradually transition into *The 3:00 PM Secret* lifestyle.

The 3:00 PM Secret 10-Day Dream Diet is a stand-alone book that builds on the philosophy of the first book while centering around a 10-day diet with menus and daily *Dream* questions. It guides you in creating a roadmap for your dream future and accelerates you into a new and healthy life. It also includes the latest research findings on how excess weight is linked to cancer and other serious diseases, a survey of healthy lifestyle practices from around the world, and Frequently Asked Questions about *The 3:00 PM Secret* lifestyle.

While working on the manuscript for *The 3:00 PM Secret: Live Slim and Strong Live Your Dreams,* I met my soulmate, David Lawrence, and we were soon married. David and I are living our dreams in Alaska and are the healthiest, strongest, and happiest we have ever been or could imagine. David has written insightful "Male Musings" throughout this book, which I believe you will find valuable and amusing. He really believes men need to pay more attention to their health. *The 3:00 PM Secret: Live Slim and Strong Live Your Dreams* also introduced Isabelle, who had successfully begun to live *The 3:00 PM Secret.* Chapter 1 and many chapter introductions of this book are written in Isabelle's voice. Isabelle and her husband, Trevor, also appear in Chapter 4 "Lifestyle Secrets and Inspirations from Alaska to the World". I hope you find her perspective fun and motivating.

PART I

Chapter 1

Is There Hope For You?
By Isabelle

A Testimonial
By Connie

Chapter 2

What The 3:00 PM Secret is

Really About

(See PART II for THE DREAM DIET)

Chapter 1

Is There Hope For You?

By Isabelle

Hi. My name is Isabelle. Debra introduced me in her book *The 3:00 PM Secret: Live Slim and Strong Live Your Dreams*. I read and followed that book, and it changed my life. I permanently solved my weight problem, rediscovered my passion for geology, met and married my soulmate, and inspired my friends to obtain the body and life of their dreams. If you read that book, you last heard from me when you read my haiku:

> At last I am free
> A body fit for my dreams
> And my destiny...
>
> Isabelle

I am here to tell you that you owe it to yourself to do *The 10-Day Dream Diet*! To start off, I'd like to share some insights I gained during my journey into *The 3:00 PM Secret*. I realized that if a person wants to be successful at weight control – and at life – he or she needs to ponder a few key questions:

(1) Am I really living the life I always dreamed about?

(2) Do I even know what I am meant to do with my life?

(3) Do I want to pursue my dream life, but don't have the confidence, energy, or strong physique I need?

(4) Am I going to spend the rest of my life **wishing** I was strong, slim, confident, and beautiful or DO something about it?

(5) Am I finally ready to become slim, strong, and empowered and to embark on my life's journey?

The last question is similar to what a sagacious friend and mentor had asked me before she launched into a painful yet life-changing diatribe of her psychoanalysis of me.

She began, "Isabelle, you're young, smart, pretty, and unhappy. What I often hear from you is that you hate the way you look. You are unable to do activities you think would be fun. You feel tired and sick a lot even though there is really nothing wrong that wouldn't dramatically improve with major weight loss and vigorous exercise. You're not getting respect or interest from men. In fact, you feel no one gives you the respect you've earned because of your weight and their prejudice that 'overweight' equals 'undisciplined'. Moreover, you've given up on your dreams. And to make matters worse, your means of comforting and nurturing yourself is to eat! You're in a downward spiral, Isabelle, and the only person who can help you is you!"

*Wow! I could not believe she would actually **say** that to me! It was totally over the top! My response was what you might expect – to defend myself, but she had heard all my excuses before.*

She went on: "Isabelle, I really care about you, and you are ruining your health and waddling into a life of debilitating and perhaps fatal diseases. You're afraid to dream, and even if you figured out what your dreams are, your body is a hindrance. But instead of ranting at you, let me offer two suggestions."

She took a drink of water, gave me a serious look, and continued, "First, stop with all the excuses and really focus on getting your body strong, slim, and healthy – you can do this Isabelle! Second, figure out how you truly want to spend the rest of your life here on Earth. You have only one chance at life, Isabelle, and the clock keeps ticking. Your dreams are worth fighting for!"

When I didn't respond, she went on. "I know I am being really hard on you, Isabelle, but trust me. I have seen too many people throw away the happiness they could have had, and even their very lives, because they refused to take control of their bodies and what goes into their mouths. They stuff down their chance of being who they could have been and having the life they could have enjoyed. Because of their failures with weight control, they lack the confidence to pursue greater dreams and give up on victories they may have achieved elsewhere in life. There is no guarantee that having a slim, strong body will make you happy and keep you disease-free, Isabelle, but carrying excess weight is a cause of many diseases you would not have had if you were slim and athletic – not to mention the psychological benefits."

Instead of wanting to clobber her for laying all this on me – which would have been perfectly reasonable – I realized she cared so much about me that she was willing to speak the truth, even if I wound up hating her for it. Instead of giving her my usual defense, I blubbered for awhile. I might add, she was blubbering along with me. I realized I was ready to **do** something, I just didn't know what. That afternoon I found *The 3:00 PM Secret: Live Slim and Strong Live Your Dreams* when I was wandering through a little bookstore searching for answers. The rest – as they say – is history. I am stronger, slimmer, and happier than I could have imagined possible.

In the following pages you will learn what to do to have the body worthy of your dreams and how to discover your dream life. Following *The 10-Day Dream Diet* is really very simple: don't eat a meal 7 to 9 hours before bedtime, eat nutritiously using the suggested menus, exercise vigorously ten minutes (or more) each day, ponder your Dream Questions and verses, and sleep 7 to 8 hours each night. That's it.

You will find as I did that when you stop eating at night and are no longer using food for comfort, nurture, or relaxation, your brain will stop associating eating with these emotional states. Then, surprisingly, you will find that your unhealthy cravings and associations with food will slowly disappear! The 3:00 PM Secret **is** the secret to permanent weight control, and pondering the Dream Questions will point you toward your dream life. I wish you much success with The 3:00 PM Secret 10-Day Dream Diet. I believe it will be a wonderful experience for you. I also hope you will be inspired to live your dreams and continue with The 3:00 PM Secret lifestyle for life. You won't regret it.

Now for some inspiration, following is a testimonial of my friend Connie's experience with The 10-Day Dream Diet.

Testimonial: Connie

The past ten years has been a struggle for me with losing and gaining weight. I would try a diet and lose weight, and then I would stop the diet and gain all the weight back plus more. I almost gave up, thinking I would have to accept that I will just be fat the rest of my life. However, I did not want to give up. Then I met Debra and had the opportunity to test *The 10-Day Dream Diet*. Debra wanted my thoughts on the food, my assessment of whether the portions were adequate, and how I would feel not eating at night. She wanted to know how I would feel while on the diet and how much weight I would lose.

After first hearing about the idea of not eating after 3:00 p.m., I expected to feel hungry and deprived the first few nights, then eventually get used to not eating dinner. To my surprise, I felt great the first nights and continued to feel good as I lost pounds. During much of *The 10-Day Dream Diet*, I was working in the yard at night and had plenty of energy! I did not feel hungry or deprived in the evenings, and when thoughts of food entered my mind, I consciously drank more water. There were two evenings when I began to feel tired and had that ever-familiar feeling that if I ate something I would feel better. On one of those evenings I drank a glass of warm milk and the other evening I ate an apple. It was enough, and I felt satisfied and perked up.

The portions set out in the plan were adequate, and I felt satisfied at each meal. Not only did I feel satisfied on the diet, but the best part was that by the end of the ten days I had lost 6.6 pounds. What a great feeling!

Day 1 of *The 10-Day Dream Diet* for me was June 17 when I weighed in at 170.8 pounds. During the first few days I was surprised how much energy I had at night! By Day 4, June 20, I was down 4 pounds to 166.8. I continued the diet while doing moderate exercise and yard work and had lots of energy. By Day 10, June 26, I weighed 164.2, down 6.6 pounds. While on the diet, I made some minor food substitutions with similar foods and ate chips and 2 cookies on Day 7 at a company picnic.

After I finished *The 10-Day Dream Diet,* I continued not eating after 3 o'clock. My meals continued to resemble the diet, though I incorporated my favorite foods. I did not, however, watch my portions. On July 15th I was happy and surprised to learn I was continuing to lose weight! That indicated to me it was not simply the portion size but the timing of my meals that was the key to my weight loss.

As I go on from this point, I intend to continue with the 3 o'clock shut off of eating, but will continue to tweak the eating plan to incorporate my favorite foods while still focusing on good nutrition. I am optimistic I can continue with my success. I think I can do this indefinitely and look forward to having weight control as an old problem I once had, but solved.

Chapter 2

What The 3:00 PM Secret is Really About

Isabelle's Insights... Hi. It's me, Isabelle, again! "So what finally motivated you to get serious and lose weight?" That was what my friend Sandy asked me when I was celebrating my weight loss and called her from Tahiti. I explained how unhappy I had been and that I just couldn't take it anymore! I was bored with my job, and I hated my body. A wise friend had helped me see my destructive and self-defeating behaviors. I told Sandy about how I wandered around a little bookstore and there it was – The 3:00 PM Secret book. I began reading it, and it seemed to speak to my soul. It said I had to make a **decision**, which I was **so** ready to do! That ingenious eating style of the 3:00 PM days really appealed to me. The doable ten-minute workout made sense, and the idea of giving myself permission to get the sleep I knew I needed was a relief. It totally resonated with me. I decided to get my life together, to honor the body God gave me, and to be free to do what my heart told me was my real life purpose – my destiny. That was it. I had begun my new journey. And the journey was wonderful! I began using my normal dinner time to explore what my life could be – to learn about what seemed interesting to me. Then I began homing in on my true, inherent interests and figuring out what steps I needed to take to live my dream life. During that time of research and discovery, I was dropping pounds and becoming strong. I began feeling healthy, optimistic, and empowered. As my life began evolving into my "dream life", the weight training and dinner skipping transformed my body into that of a slim, strong athlete. I felt I was finally living the life I was meant to live.

2.1. MAKING A DECISION ABOUT YOUR DREAM LIFE

Are you unhappy with your life and stuffing down your disappointments? You need to focus your attention on investigating what you truly **want** to do with your life! What if there were questions that could reveal your life's dreams? As you go through the ten-day diet, you will answer your *dream* questions each day.

Have you ever really pondered what you would *really* love to do with your time? Do you know what is truly important to you? There was a time when I was so out of touch with myself that I could not answer these kinds of questions. I had to really think – "What **am** I really interested in?" To answer that question, I spent time looking through magazines on subjects in which I had some interest. I paid attention to what articles I wound up reading all the way through. What most intrigued me? What did I most enjoy doing with my time? What gave me optimistic feelings toward the future? What was my calling? Now let me ask you – can you give yourself the mental time to become immersed in the possibilities of your life?

Are there one or more fields that especially interest you? Find sources of information on these subjects and begin learning. See if you actually read all the information and if it holds your attention. If it does, that's a pretty good clue you should invest time learning more. Once you discover your primary areas of inherent interest, integrate them into your life as hobbies. See where it leads.

It may take time and exploration to ascertain your passion and purpose. It is a process. If you want God's guidance, you need to focus on your walk with Him so you will be sensitive to His sometimes subtle nudges.   Once you discover what you feel passionate about, you can begin to reorder your life so as to immerse yourself in what you truly love and value. You can embark on a new journey, turning your true interests into a life-long adventure.

Make a conscious decision not to live a life of unfulfilled dreams that you stuff down with food! The truth is, the only person who can stop you from being exactly what you want to be and having the life you desire is you. You need your body to assist you in living your dream life. As you proceed in determining what your dream life looks like, you can use *The 3:00 PM Secret* to attain and maintain your dream body. Then, you can fully experience the life you were meant to live.

2.2. OBESITY AND DISEASE

Obesity and disease – now there's a happy subject! That's right, it's me, Isabelle, again. Before Debra lays this really important, yet scary, info on you, let me just say that if you take it to heart, it can save your future and your life. You really need to know about this, so you can truly understand the direct consequences of your behaviors and choices. Do you really want to live a life marked with illness, medical treatments, restrictions, and immobility if you can possibly avoid some or most of it? Why? So you can shove food into your mouth at will? That's not freedom, it's bondage! If you want to live fully, please stop killing yourself with bad habits. Sorry to be so blunt, but like my sagacious friend said, "Isabelle, I really care about you and you are ruining your health and waddling into a life of debilitating and perhaps fatal diseases..." Please, care about yourself and those who love you and create a strong, healthy, slim body. What I have found is that just knowing the facts on lifestyle and disease motivates me to avoid junk food and get out and run even when the weather is terrible! And what's more, once you get free of bad foods and a sedentary life, you won't miss it!

New research findings linking excess weight with various diseases are alarming! I am persuaded that carrying excess weight is a health time bomb. Toxins are stored in fat cells, and having excess fat cells in your body creates a toxic environment. People who are overweight or obese are more likely to develop heart disease, stroke, high blood pressure, diabetes, gallbladder disease, gout, sleep apnea, osteoarthritis, and many types of cancer. That's the bad news. The good news is that you have the power to increase your chances of living a healthy, vital life.

While heart disease, cancer, and stroke are the three leading causes of death in the U.S., cancer is the disease that people worry about the most. In November 2007 a *Landmark Report* was published by the American Institute for Cancer Research (AICR) and the World Cancer Research Fund (WCRF) on cancer. The report, called *"Food, Nutrition, Physical Activity, and the Prevention of Cancer: a Global Perspective"* is the most comprehensive ever published. (The report can be viewed at www.dietandcancerreport.org.)

The *Report* confirms that cancer is caused by being overweight or obese and that **excess body fat causes cancer**. While there are other causes of cancer such as tobacco use, infectious agents, medication, radiation, industrial chemicals, and carcinogenic agents in food and drink, the one cause that we have total control over is our own weight. The authors of the *Report* estimated that cancer cases worldwide would be *cut by one-third* if people would follow their prescribed diet and exercise advice, *especially maintaining a weight at the low end of the "normal" BMI[1] range*. It is a mystery to me why the results of this report have not been prominently reported.

The *Report* involved teams of scientists from around the world, hundreds of peer reviewers, and 21 international experts. They reviewed over 7,000 large studies on diet, physical activity, and weight, and their effect on 17 different cancers. The report revealed that excess body fat increases risk for numerous cancers. Another important finding of the *Report* was that **consuming red meat and processed meat causes cancer**.

One of the Panel members, Dr. James, said "The most striking finding in the report is that **excess body fat increases risk for numerous cancers**. That is why *body weight is the focus of our first recommendation."* He also said, *"Even small amounts of excess body fat, especially if carried at the waist, increase risk."* He further stated, "Cancer is preventable. There are changes you can make in your daily life that will reduce your chances of developing cancer." The *Report* also noted that cancer risk increases in a dose response manner with body weight so that *for additional pounds, the risk increases.*

---

[1] BMI is Body Mass Index. See Appendix 2.

According to the *Report*, body fat is convincingly linked to six cancers and suggestive in others. Following is a brief summary of the *Report's* findings on the cancers having the strongest links:

Colon and Rectum: "The evidence that body fatness is a *cause* of this cancer is convincing." ***Red meat (beef, pork, and lamb) and processed meats (bacon, ham, sausage, and lunchmeat) were found to be direct causes of colorectal cancer.*** (*Every 1.7 ounces of processed meat consumed per day increases risk of colorectal cancer by 21 percent!*) Heavy alcohol consumption (in men) and abdominal fatness also are causes of this cancer. Colorectal cancer is the third most common cancer worldwide. It is fatal in almost half of cases and is the fourth most common cause of death from cancer. Physical activity helps protect against colorectal cancer.

Kidney: "The evidence that body fatness is a *cause* of this cancer is convincing." It is the fifteenth most common cancer worldwide with an average 5-year survival rate around 50%. Smoking is also a *cause* of kidney cancer.

Pancreas: "The evidence that body fatness is a *cause* of this cancer is convincing." It is the thirteenth most common cancer worldwide and is almost always fatal.

Endometrium: "The evidence that body fatness is a *cause* of this cancer is convincing." Abdominal fatness is also a particular *cause*. It is the eighth most common cancer in women. Around 75% of women with this cancer survive for 5 years. Physical activity is believed to help protect against this cancer.

Post-menopausal breast cancer: "The evidence that body fatness is a *cause* of this cancer is convincing." Abdominal body fatness is probably also a cause. Breast cancer is the most common cancer in women worldwide. It is fatal in under half of all cases, but is the leading cause of death from cancer in women. Physical activity is believed to help protect against post-menopausal breast cancer and may also help protect against pre-menopausal breast cancer.

Adenocarcinoma of the Esophagus: "The evidence that body fatness is a *cause* of this cancer is convincing." It is the eighth most common type of cancer worldwide and is usually fatal. (Please note that there are two common types of esophageal cancer, adenocarcinoma and squamous cell carcinoma.)

Cancer of the Gallbladder: "Body fatness is probably a cause of cancer of the gallbladder, and people with gallstones are more likely to develop gallbladder cancer."

The *Report's* Recommendations for Cancer Prevention are:

1. *Be as lean as possible* within the normal range of body weight.
2. *Be physically active* as part of everyday life.
3. *Limit* consumption of energy-dense foods. *Avoid sugary drinks*.
4. *Eat mostly foods of plant origin*. (5 or more servings of vegetables and fruit daily)
5. *Limit intake of red meat and avoid processed meat*.
6. Limit alcoholic drinks.
7. Limit consumption of salt.
   Avoid moldy cereals (grains) or pulses (legumes).
8. Aim to meet nutritional needs through diet alone.
9. Breastfeed.
10. Cancer survivors should follow these recommendations.

So, how does body fatness cause cancer? The Report explains that body fat influences the levels of certain hormones and growth factors, creating an environment that encourages cancer growth. Levels of insulin, insulin-like growth factors, leptin, and estrogens are all elevated in overweight people and can promote the growth of cancer cells. Fat tissue is the main site of estrogen synthesis in men and postmenopausal women. Elevated levels of sex hormones are strongly associated with risk of postmenopausal breast and endometrial cancers and possibly colon and other cancers. Insulin resistance is also increased by body fatness, especially abdominal fatness, resulting in the pancreas compensating by increasing insulin production. This hyperinsulinaemia increases the risk of certain cancers. The increased insulin and Insulin Growth Factor-1 levels that accompany body fatness result in increased estradiol (natural estrogen) in men and women. Body fat also stimulates the body's inflammatory response, which may contribute to the initiation and progression of several cancers.

In summary, the authors of the AICR and WCRF *Report* suggest we could cut worldwide cancer cases by one-third by following their guidelines. But what does it mean to cut cancer cases by one-third? Searching medical and U.S. government cancer websites reveals you have about a 40% chance of developing cancer during your life. That means for every 100 people, 40 of them are likely to develop cancer. If we all follow the *Report's* advice and subsequently cut cancer cases by about one-third, this would leave us as a group with only about a 27% chance of developing cancer.[2] (I'd rather be in the 27% group.)

There are other scary diseases such as *dementia and Alzheimer's disease that are also linked with excess body fat and being overweight.* A large survey of studies concluded that having an elevated BMI significantly increases a person's risk of dementia.[3] A 27-year study of 10,276 people showed obese people (BMI ≥30) had a *74% increased risk of developing dementia*, while overweight people (BMI 25-29.9) had a *35% greater risk of developing dementia*.[4] Yikes! Another study revealed that women who are overweight at age 70 had an increased risk of developing Alzheimer's disease, and that for every 1.0 unit increase in BMI at age 70 years, Alzheimer's disease risk increased by an astounding 36%![5] Even people who are not significantly overweight are at increased risk of developing dementia and Alzheimer's disease if they carry excess abdominal fat.[6]

Obesity is also linked to high blood pressure, which increases your risk of developing cardiovascular diseases and can cause long-term damage to your heart, blood vessels, and kidneys. Even moderate weight gain is associated with an increased risk of developing high blood pressure. Not surprisingly, treatment for high blood pressure includes weight loss and regular physical activity.[7] High blood pressure is one of the leading causes of kidney failure. People with kidney failure must either endure dialysis or receive a kidney transplant to stay alive.[8]

As your weight increases, your chances of having two or more of the following also increase: *Type II diabetes mellitus, gallbladder disease, coronary heart disease, high blood cholesterol level, high blood pressure, and osteoarthritis.*[9] Being overweight in middle age significantly increases your risk

---

[2] http://seer.cancer.gov/statfacts/html/all.html; http://surveillance.cancer.gov/statistics/types/lifetime_risk.html; http://www.cancer.org/docroot/CRI/content/CRI_2_6x_Lifetime_Probability_of_Developing_or_Dying_From_Cancer.asp

[3] Age and Ageing v.36, No.1, p.23-29, January 2007

[4] British Medical Journal v.330, p.1360, 6/11/05

[5] Archives of Internal Medicine v.163, p.1524, 2003

[6] Neurology. R. A. Whitmer PhD, online Mar 26, 2008 (Neurology 2008, doi:10.1212/01.wnl.0000306313.89165.ef)

[7] American Journal of Physiology-Regulatory, Integrative, and Comparative Physiology, May 2004

[8] http://kidney.niddk.nih.gov/kudiseases/pubs/highblood, NIDDK is part of the National Institutes of Health

[9] Journal of the American Medical Association v.282, p.1523-1529, 1999

of *severe cardiovascular disease, coronary heart disease, strokes, diabetes, and kidney problems* later in life.[10] If a child is overweight, particularly as an older child, the risk of having *blocked coronary arteries and heart disease* as an adult increases.[11] *Being overweight or obese, especially at younger ages, substantially increases the lifetime risk of developing diabetes.*[12]

Excess body weight during midlife is associated with **increasing the risk of premature death** by 20% to 40% among overweight persons and by 200% to 300% or more among obese persons.[13]

What if we use an airplane analogy for the effects of excess body fat on several of the overweight and obesity related ailments? Imagine that Alzheimer's disease is the airplane's right wing, cancer is the left wing, cardiovascular disease is the tail, and diabetes is the computer guidance system. Being overweight is analogous to increasing your risk by somewhere between 10% and 30% that any one of these airplane systems would malfunction or fall off during your flight.

Suppose you get on an airplane, fasten your seatbelt, and then hear the pilot announce that during the flight this airplane has a 10% to 30% chance of losing a wing, tail, or guidance system, and therefore crashing. Are you going to remain on that airplane? Can you imagine anyone flying in an airplane with those odds? Yet the same person will create a body that gives them similar or worse odds for developing at least one of the following: cancer, diabetes, heart disease, stroke, or Alzheimer's disease.

The rewards of weight control, exercise, and living healthfully not only include having a more vital life in a beautiful, strong body, but also increase your chances of living longer with a healthy mind and body. While there are no

---

[10] Journal of the American Medical Association v.295, No.2, p.190-198, 1/11/06; Annals of Internal Medicine v.144, No.1, p.21-28, 1/3/06; Science News, v.169, No.2, p.21, 1/14/06

[11] New England Journal of Medicine v.357, No.23, p.2329, 12/6/07; Science News, v.172, No.24, p.381, 12/15/07

[12] Diabetes Care v.30, p.1562-1566, 2007

[13] The New England Journal of Medicine v.355, No.8, p.763-778, 8/24/06

guarantees of perfect health, being slim, fit, and strong can reduce disease risk and aid in a speedier recovery from illnesses.

2.3. THE 3:00 PM SECRET

Definition, Benefits, and Why it Works

Isabelle continues... *I still remember what my friend, Josie, said when I told her that a big key to my weight loss success was that I simply don't eat much after 3:00 PM most days. I told her I was surprised to discover I really was not hungry until breakfast. Josie was shocked! I insisted that for the first time in I could not remember how many years I had time for myself at night rather than that old prepare, eat, clean up, get ready for bed routine. And I had so much energy!*

I explained I was going 16 hours from my last meal until breakfast, with the last 8 hours being asleep, while Josie, a breakfast skipper, was trying to go 18 hours from dinner to lunch with the last several hours attempting to work while struggling with low energy. Of course, Josie always wound up eating a mid-morning Danish, along with her usual feeding frenzy at night.

That was before Josie tried The 3:00 PM Secret for herself. Today, she is slim, strong, and beautiful! She has a confidence she says she never had before, which helped her begin living her dream life. For her, that means traveling all over the world! Now every time I hear from her she is in some new and exotic place! My friends thought The 3:00 PM Secret was some kind of fad diet – but it's not. It is a permanent lifestyle which I love. Once I went through the period of transitioning away from eating late in my day, I discovered many benefits to The 3:00 PM Secret beyond being a reliable method of weight control and reducing the risk of diseases. I found my dream life.

The 3:00 PM Secret Definition

The 3:00 PM Secret involves (1) Pursuing your dream life; (2) Refraining from eating a meal 7 to 9 hours before bedtime; (3) Eating nutritiously; (4) Exercising vigorously at least ten minutes each day; and (5) Sleeping 7 to 8 hours each night. In addition, (6) *The 10-Day Dream Diet* asks you to cogitate on a *Dream* question each day to help you discover your dream life.

The 3:00 PM Secret Benefits

(1) Imagine being cured of emotional eating. By eating early when you need food and not eating in the evening, your brain begins to associate eating with nutrition rather than nurture. You will stop looking to food to fill emotional needs.

(2) *The 3:00 PM Secret* lifestyle gives you energy during the day when you most need it. Your body has the remainder of the day and night to burn what you have eaten. People who follow *The 3:00 PM Secret* also report having more energy at night – they have more overall energy.

(3) Have you ever wished you had more free time? *The 3:00 PM Secret* lifestyle gives you more free time at night to do what is ultimately more important and interesting than preparing, eating, and cleaning up a meal you did not need.

(4) You will find you have changed your perspective away from a food-centered life to a life focused on your dreams and purposes. You will feel hopeful and optimistic!

(5) Eating at night will be unattractive to you – and you will feel overfull when you do. This makes it easy to continue in this lifestyle and effortlessly maintain your slim, strong body. Once you integrate *The 3:00 PM Secret* into your life, you will never consider going back to night eating!

(6) It supports the primary lifestyle treatment guidelines for reducing gastroesophageal reflux disease (GERD), which are to avoid eating at night or within three to four hours of bedtime or lying down[14] and to lose weight.[15]

---

[14] http://www.gastromd.com/education/gerd.html;
http://www.clevelandclinic.org/health/health-info/docs/1600/1697.asp?index=7042&src=news;
http://www.gicare.com/pated/ecdgs39.htm

[15] American Journal of Gastroenterology v.102, No.10, p.2128-34, October 2007

The 3:00 PM Secret Why It Works?

Do you think the time of day when you eat really matters? The first *3:00 PM Secret* book, *The 3:00 PM Secret: Live Slim and Strong Live Your Dreams,* explained why front-loading your calories earlier in the day and not eating at night is so effective. The idea is to eat your food early in the day, so the calories you consume can be burned for energy while you are active. Having a healthy, nutritious breakfast and lunch provides fuel to carry you through your day when you need energy and can burn what you eat. It is very logical. Not eating a meal late in your day or at night allows you to burn what you ate earlier in the day and not store it as fat while you relax and sleep.

Have you ever wondered how Sumo wrestlers gain and maintain their high weights? Since ancient times Sumo wrestlers have perfected the ability to become very fat. Their livelihoods depend on it! How do they do it? They fast throughout the morning while they are exercising, eat a huge lunch, and then nap several hours immediately after eating, which is crucial to their weight gain. After the afternoon nap, they may do further, though less rigorous, exercise, and then have their last large meal at night.

Successful weight gain by Sumo wrestlers is credited to the large quantity of food eaten during their afternoon and evening meals in conjunction with the lack of activity after meals during digestion.[16] Sound familiar – the typical American lifestyle! Skipping breakfast makes them hungrier so they can eat more. *It is believed that overeating late in the day causes a drop in metabolism and encourages the body to store fat.* After meals, Sumo wrestlers sleep so most of the calories they eat will be deposited as fat.[17] These guys are experts on being fat. Isn't it worth considering the wisdom they have developed over the centuries and applying it to *weight loss*? It seems that without realizing it, overweight Westerners have adopted Sumo eating habits, except we fail to mimic Sumo's daily exercise.

---

[16] The Wave Magazine Banzai Appetite; November 2002 issue of Saveur Magazine; http://www.pbs.org/independentlens/sumoeastandwest/sumo.html; http://oldeee.see.ed.ac.uk/~njt/Japanese/sumo.pdf

[17] http://www.discoverychannelasia.com/sumo/become_a_sumo_wrestler/index.shtml,Copyright © 2007 Discovery Comm. Inc

So, is when you eat as important as what you eat? "A number of recent studies in animals linking energy regulation and the circadian clock at the molecular, physiological, and behavioral levels raise the possibility that *the timing of food intake itself may play a significant role in weight gain.*" In a new study, mice that ate when they should have been asleep gained more weight than mice that ate at normal hours during their "day". A control group of mice were fed during their normal awake time. Another group ate the same meals during their sleep time, which disrupts the body's normal 24-hour circadian rhythm. After six weeks, the off-schedule mice weighed almost 20% more than the controls, supporting the idea that consuming calories when you should be sleeping is harmful. Researchers suggest there is more to weight than calories,[18] providing more evidence that timing matters.

In fact, evidence is mounting that front-loading your calories early in the day is an excellent way to control weight. A study of 6,764 people ages 40 to 75 found those who ate the most in the morning gained the least amount of weight. The study suggests that a redistribution of daily *calorie* intake, so that *more calories are consumed at breakfast and fewer calories are consumed later in the day,* may help to reduce weight gain in middle-aged adults."[19]

Another study compared meal patterns of lean and obese women. It found that *obese women ate a larger number of meals later in the day,* consuming fewer calories in the morning and a greater portion of total calories in the afternoon and evening/night.[20] Researchers have found that *skipping breakfast* is associated with increased prevalence of obesity.[21] Overweight people often skip breakfast, which means they eat more later in the day and at night. In fact, one study showed that overweight people who were trying to diet tended to eat little or no breakfast, a light lunch, and consumed most of their calories late in the day and at night. Conversely, people who successfully lost weight ate breakfast.[22] Another study revealed that the more food people consumed in the morning, the fewer total calories they ate for that day, whereas when people ate their meals in

[18] http://sciencenow.sciencemag.org/cgi/content/full/2009/903/1; ScienceNOW Daily News, Kean, 3 September 2009; Obesity (2009) doi:10.1038/oby.2009.264

[19] American Journal of Epidemiology v.167, No.2 p.188-192, 1/15/08

[20] European Journal of Clinical Nutrition v.56, No.8 p.740-747 August 2002

[21] American Journal of Epidemiology v.158, No.1, p. 85-92, 7/1/03

[22] January-February 2002, U.S. Food and Drug administration

the afternoon and evening, they ate more total calories.[23] Participants in a study who made the most substantial changes in eating habits to comply with a diet program were found to achieve better results, and breakfast eating reduced dietary fat intake and impulsive snacking.[24] *The 3:00 PM Secret* lifestyle could certainly be considered a "substantial change".

An analysis of *National Health and Nutrition Examination* surveys from 1971 to 2004 found breakfast skipping to be one of the three critical factors that appear to contribute to obesity in young people.[25] Another 5-year study of weight change in 2,216 adolescents found that while breakfast eaters consumed more calories than breakfast skippers, they had lower BMI's, were leaner, and were more physically active, suggesting they had more energy and burned off more of what they ate. These breakfast eaters also ate more nutritiously.[26]

Consuming a lot at night has also been linked with psychological problems, classified as "night-eating syndrome". Night-eating syndrome has been attributed to those who consume more than half of their total daily calories after 7:00 p.m., skip breakfast at least 4 days per week, and often have difficulty falling asleep or staying asleep. People with night-eating syndrome have been shown to lose less weight on weight-loss programs and have more depression and low self-esteem.[27] Night-eating syndrome was first characterized in 1955 as morning anorexia (appetite loss), evening hyperphagia (excessive overeating), and insomnia.[28] Obese people are more likely than non-obese people to have this syndrome.[29] Also, night-eating syndrome increases in prevalence with increasing obesity[30] High rates of the night-eating syndrome have been found in obese patients in bariatric (obesity) surgery clinics.[31] Night-eating syndrome is

[23] Journal of Nutrition 134, p.104-111, January 2004, The American Society for Nutritional Sciences

[24] American Journal of Clinical Nutrition, v.55, p.645, 1992

[25] Journal of the American Medical Association v.295, No.20, p.2385 –2393, 2006

[26] Pediatrics v. 121, No.3, p.e638-e645, March 2008

[27] Obesity Research v.9, p.264, 2001; The North American Association for the Study of Obesity

[28] American Journal of Medicine v.19, No.1, p.78-86, 1955

[29] Am J Psychiatry v.163, p156, January 2006

[30] JAMA v.282, No.7, p657, 8/18/99

[31] Int J Eat Dis v.19, p.23, 1996/ Obesity Research v.12, p.1789, 2004

associated with obesity and depressed mood.[32] A study of patients with either Type I or II diabetes revealed that those with night-eating behaviors were more likely to be obese and have emotional problems.[33]

Clearly, the timing of when we eat, with respect to when we sleep and when we are active, matters. In fact, the idea of inserting time intervals between meals has been receiving a lot of attention in the area of intermittent fasting. Research on intermittent fasting has been associated with studies of calorie restriction since the benefits are similar. Both caloric restriction and intermittent fasting, while maintaining vitamin and mineral intake, can extend lifespan, increase disease resistance, and have profound effects on brain function and its resistance to injury and disease.

In animal studies, researchers found that intermittent fasting resulted in an increase in the production of brain-derived neurotrophic factor, which makes neurons in the brain more resistant to dysfunction and degeneration.[34] Increasing the time interval between meals, such as 20 to 24 hours, has been shown to have beneficial effects on the brain and overall health of mice that are independent of how many calories the mice ate. There is substantial evidence that controlled calorie restriction and intermittent fasting can increase lifespan and protect various tissues against disease,[35] and researchers are looking at these as potential anticancer strategies.[36] In a study on humans, healthy young men practiced intermittent fasting on every second day for 20 hour periods for 15 days, and it was found that intermittent fasting increased insulin sensitivity in fat and other tissues. The researchers determined that these cycles of eating and fasting led to improvements in metabolic function.[37] Moreover, intermittent fasting and caloric restriction have been shown to extend lifespan and increase resistance to age-related diseases in rodents and monkeys and improve the health of overweight humans. Both intermittent fasting and caloric restriction enhance cardiovascular and brain functions and improve several risk factors for coronary artery disease

---

[32] The Journal of Clinical Endocrinology & Metabolism v.90, No.11, 6214, 2005

[33] Diabetes Care v.29, p1800, 2006

[34] Annual Reviews of Nutrition v.25, p.237, 2005

[35] Journal of Neurochemistry v.84, No.3, p.417-31, Feb 2003; Ageing Research Reviews v.7, No.1, p.43-8, Jan 2008

[36] Carcinogenesis v.23, No.5, p.817-822, May 2002

[37] Journal of Applied Physiology, v.99, p.2128-2136, 2005

and stroke including a reduction in blood pressure and increased insulin sensitivity.[38]

The 3:00 PM Secret 10-Day Dream Diet is *not* an intermittent fasting program since, by definition, intermittent fasting generally suggests 20 to 24 hours of fasting. Nevertheless, the concept of using intermittent fasts to improve health is compatible with *The 3:00 PM Secret* lifestyle, which offers shorter periods of 15 to 16 hours without a meal beginning in the afternoon and ending with breakfast. Commercial advocates of intermittent fasting often suggest beginning a fast at bedtime and fasting throughout the morning into the afternoon and beyond. This produces behaviors similar to breakfast skipping and results in not having food energy during your day *when you need it*, followed by excessive eating at night (when you don't need food energy) once the fast is terminated. In addition, while *The 3:00 PM Secret* is *not* a lifestyle of calorie restriction, people following *The 3:00 PM Secret* will find they have lost their unhealthy cravings for excessive calorie intake – that is one of the wonderful rewards of this lifestyle!

If you want to lose weight and maintain a healthy, low weight, then simply eat nutritiously and early, don't eat in the afternoon and evening, exercise daily, get enough sleep, and live your dream life!

So, why do people think they need to eat at night? The desire to eat at night or when you really don't need food can come from cultural tradition, habit, boredom, or a need for emotional nurturing. Food is really for maximizing nutrition and making your body healthy and strong – not for pleasure, nurture, or filling time. It is not that difficult to turn a preoccupation with food into a hope-filled life of pursuing your dreams.

---

[38] Journal of Nutritional Biochemistry v.16, No.3, p.129-37, Mar 2005

* *

MALE MUSING ON TEMPTATION

Don't Resist the Temptation - Remove It!

Have you ever found yourself biting into an unhealthy treat, when you stopped for an instant and thought, "I wasn't going to eat this!" and then continued eating it anyway? Have you found yourself rummaging around your kitchen for a snack just because you don't know what else to do? Have you tried to resist eating some forbidden food for a day or two, only to finally give in and stuff a lot of it into your mouth? If so, congratulations! You're fully human! It is a rare person who can resist a favorite food when it is offered or is resting nearby, calling out in an ethereal but insistent voice, "I'm here. Come and eat me."

Inevitably, after your latest culinary sin, you beat yourself up for being so weak. Your food demon helps out by encouraging you to give up on whatever weight loss diet you happen to be on since you're obviously hopeless.

Maybe you get back with the program for a while, but eventually you fail one time too many. Besides, you really **do** enjoy eating a lot of certain unhealthy foods. So, sooner or later, you're back where you started, except you've lost a little more faith in yourself, and your hope for getting your weight under control is further tarnished and diminished.

Where did you go wrong? Didn't it all start with just a few small nibbles that you took without really intending or wanting to? Unless you can transplant a new self-control center into your brain, you have a problem. Is there an achievable solution? Yes. Think about it. Your food cravings and temptations ebb and flow. They do not gnaw at you 24/7 but just during periodic bouts of weakness, hunger, or emotional upset. Those moments do not last forever, and that's the key to the solution.

What if at the very moment your weak side was looking for the food you really don't want to eat, the tempting food simply was not there? What if the cookies, candy, ice cream, or chips were not even in the house? What if the huge tin of nuts or bag of donuts did not exist?

If you had to put on a coat, leave the house, and drive to the store to get the forbidden food you were craving, isn't it possible that you wouldn't go to all the trouble or that, by the time you got to the store, you would have retaken control of your hands and mouth?

You will find it far easier not to eat the foods that have a hold on you, but that you really don't want to consume, if you move the battle line from your mouth or your pantry all the way out the door, down the driveway, down the street, and inside your food store.

It will be easier to fight off the certifiably bad foods that try to jump into your cart if you go there with a carefully-drawn list and stay out of the junk food aisles altogether. You may not win every battle, but you don't need to be perfect. If you cannot keep garbage out of your cart, then either have a friend or family member shop for you or take along an accountability friend.

Removing temptation from the home was very important for me in changing eating habits. Now, after living the healthy 3PM lifestyle for several years, my cravings for bad foods are gone. In fact, when I eat unhealthy foods, overeat, or eat late, I do not feel good. I found that eventually my mind was reprogrammed to **like** healthy living.

Also beware of friends or relatives who unconsciously sabotage your efforts by waving your favorite treats in front of you. They may feel sorry for you because you're trying to eat healthy and eat less. They may even feel guilty they're not doing the same. Unlike bad foods, you can't banish these friends and family members from your home and life. But you can thank them for their well-intentioned gesture and then refuse the treat or limit your intake at the unhealthy meal. Then you can enlist them to help you achieve your goals by ending their misguided food ministry. After your tenth request to cease the sabotage, it will begin to dawn on them that you're really serious. When you are firm and respect yourself and your eating goals, they will respect you too. You never know – you may even inspire them to follow your lead, especially when they see you getting healthier, slimmer, stronger, and happier.

* * * * * * * * * * * * * * * * * * *

2.4. TEN NUTRITION TIPS

Isabelle continues... Hi. It's me, Isabelle, again. I remember when my husband, Trevor, first told me that wild animals possess an amazing ability to select a diet that meets their nutritional requirements, and yet they avoid eating significant amounts of poisonous or toxic substances. I must have realized this, but I had never really thought about it before that moment – standing in the library the first time I laid eyes on Trevor. I was hooked. He went on to say that somehow wild animals can recognize a food's nutritional value (even though God didn't put labels on them), which is not necessarily related to the food's taste or smell. Then, I asked him, "Do you think we possess this instinctive ability as well?" With that question, Trevor thought I was smart!

Do we instinctively possess the ability to know whether a food is nutritious or toxic? It *is* a thought-provoking question, particularly because we humans frequently overeat non-nutritious, unhealthy, manufactured "foods", while under-eating nutritious, healthy, natural, unprocessed foods. This often leads to obese yet somewhat malnourished bodies. In fact, eating junk food has been shown to elicit addictive behavior and compulsive eating leading to obesity in rats.[39] It is best to stay away from junk food from the start and avoid feeling addicted. If you already have a problem, get yourself free and after some time away, junk foods will no longer have control over you.

If we provide our bodies with optimum nutrition while not overeating, we can positively affect our health and lifespan. People in certain cultures have better health and longer lifespans than others. It is believed that dietary habits play a large role. Diets from the healthiest cultures include an emphasis on vegetables, unsaturated fats in the form of fish and olive oil, fruits, soy, and whole grains, as well as a de-emphasis on sugar, processed foods, meat, and dairy. There are also bonus foods, such as mineral-rich seaweeds, garlic, ginger, wine, omega-3-rich oils such as flaxseed oil and fish oil, green tea, and turmeric.

---

[39] Science News v.176, No.11, p.8, 11/21/09

Curcumin in the spice, *turmeric*, is being studied for its potential anti-inflammatory, anti-cancer, and anti-tumor benefits,[40] as well as its possible protective qualities against cataract formation[41] and Alzheimer's disease.[42] Omega-3 fatty acids found in fish oil and flaxseed oil are also being studied for their efficacy in preventing and treating Alzheimer's disease and dementia. The omega-3 fatty acid docosahexaenoic acid (DHA) was shown to increase the production of a protein, LR11, which destroys the characteristic plaques found in the brains of Alzheimer's patients.[43] A large study of adults over age 65 found that those who regularly consumed omega-3 rich oils considerably cut their risk of dementia and Alzheimer's disease, and that people who ate fruits and vegetables daily significantly cut their risk of dementia. These results suggest that a diet rich in fish, omega-3 oils, fruits, and vegetables can lower the risk of dementia and Alzheimer's disease.[44] High dietary intake of omega-3 fatty acids has also been strongly linked to lower rates of cardiovascular disease. Fish oil supplements lower triglyceride levels and may also prevent arrhythmias, reduce inflammation, inhibit platelet aggregation, and lower blood pressure – all of which should reduce cardiovascular risk.[45] It was even reported recently that a diet rich in omega-3 fatty acids may delay the onset of Type I juvenile-onset diabetes in children prone to the disease.[46] Omega-3 oils have been studied for their many health benefits and should be part of your daily diet.

Emphasizing plant foods in your diet can have a positive impact on your health. Fruits and vegetables, with their abundance of vitamins, minerals, phytochemicals, free-radical fighting antioxidants, and other beneficial compounds can fight off diseases, enhance health, protect neurons from free radicals, and help give us longer, healthier lives. Foods that fight free radicals

---

[40] Carcinogenesis, v.20, No.5, p.911, May 1999; Carcinogenesis v.14, p.493, 1993 by Oxford University Press; American Journal of Clinical Nutrition v.70, No.3, p.491, September 1999; Science News, v.166, No.15, p.238, 10/9/04

[41] American Journal of Clinical Nutrition v.64, 761, 1996; Investigative Ophthalmology Visual Science, v.46, No.6, p.2092, June 2005

[42] The Journal of Neuroscience v.21, No.21, p.8370, 11/1/01; Current Alzheimer Research v.2, p.131-136, 2005; BBC NEWS, 11/21/01 http://news.bbc.co.uk/2/hi/health/1668932.stm; Annals of Indian Academy of Neurology v.11, No.1, p.13-19, 2008; Proceedings of the International Academy of Sciences v.104, No.31, p.12849, 7/31/07; Science News, v.172, No.3, p.37, 7/21/07; Science News, v.172, No.11, p.167, 9/15/07

[43] Journal of Neuroscience v.27, No.52, p.14299 - 14307 12/26/07

[44] Neurology, v.69, p.1921-1930, 11/13/07

[45] Cleveland Clinic Journal of Medicine v.76, No.4, p.245-51, April 2009

[46] Journal of the American Medical Association v.298, No.12, p.1420, 9/26/07; Science News, v.172, No.15, p.237, 10/13/07

have health-promoting, anti-aging benefits.[47] It has been shown that a high consumption of plant-based foods such as fruits, vegetables, nuts, and whole grains is associated with a significantly lower risk of coronary artery disease and stroke.[48] In the *Report* on cancer discussed earlier in this chapter we learned that red meats and processed meats *cause* colon cancer. It makes sense that vegetarians not only tend to weigh less than non-vegetarians, but also have a lower incidence of certain diseases such as heart disease, high blood pressure, certain cancers, and diabetes,[49] particularly Type II diabetes.[50]

The benefits of plant foods as well as omega-3 fatty acids, turmeric, exercise, and curbing calories are well documented.[51] Everything you eat or drink goes into your body and affects it in either a positive or negative way.

The following are easy guidelines for optimum nutrition.

The Ten Nutrition Tips

1. ***Eat vegetables daily*** such as spinach, broccoli, chard, kale, purple cabbage, cauliflower, onions, garlic, parsley, red and green peppers, and other highly colored vegetables. If you do not eat vegetables daily, at least drink fresh vegetable juices.

2. ***Eat fruit daily*** such as grapefruit, blueberries, strawberries, apricots, tangerines, apples, lemons, oranges, figs, raspberries, peaches, plums, cantaloupe, cherries, pears, grapes, and kiwis. If you do not eat fruit daily, drink fresh, low-sugar fruit juices.

3. ***Consume omega-3 essential fatty acids daily***. The most concentrated sources of *omega-3* fatty acids include fatty and cold-water fish such as salmon and tuna, flaxseed oil, fish oil supplements, and omega-3 fatty acid supplements. Additional sources of omega-3 fatty acids include pumpkin seeds, walnuts, and flaxseeds. High quality sources of *omega-6*

---

[47] Nature v.408, No.6809, p.239, 11/9/00
[48] American Journal of Clinical Nutrition,v.78, No.3, p.544, September 2003
[49] Nutrition Reviews v.64, No.4, p.175, April 2006
[50] Am J Clin Nutr. v.78, No.3 Suppl, p.610, Sept 2003
[51] Science News, v.169, No.9, p.136, 3/4/06

fatty acids may be consumed in lesser amounts. These can be found in health-food stores and include evening primrose oil, borage oil, black currant seed oil, and gooseberry oils. Additional healthy sources of *omega-6* fatty acids include raw nuts and seeds, legumes, leafy green vegetables, and grains. Note that common vegetable oils such as corn, safflower, sunflower, soybean, cottonseed, and sesame contain omega-6 fatty acids; however, these oils are generally processed and hydrogenated and should be avoided because they contain harmful transfats. It is recommended that we consume a balance of omega-6 and omega-3-rich foods, yet omega-6-rich foods are far more prevalent, so we need to pay attention to getting enough omega-3 rich foods. The *monounsaturated fatty acids* also have tremendous health benefits and should be included in your diet. Good sources of monounsaturated fatty acids include ~~olive oil,~~ avocados, and nuts.

4. *Consume healthy protein*, which can be obtained from various foods including fish and seafood such as salmon and tuna, nuts, seeds, nut and seed butters, soybeans, tempeh, miso, tofu, beans, legumes, ~~wheat germ,~~ sprouted beans and grains, organic yogurt, and ~~limited amounts of~~ animal protein such as organic cottage cheese and eggs.

   Avoid glutens + oils. Eat eggs. KARL 2016

5. *Choose whole-food complex carbohydrates* such as black, pinto, navy, and lima beans; split peas; legumes; lentils; basmati; brown rice; wild rice; ~~oats;~~ unprocessed whole grains including buckwheat, millet, amaranth, spelt, quinoa, ~~barley, rye, bulgur, and whole-grain pumpernickel;~~ sprouts from vegetables, sunflowers, beans, and grains; and, if you are not sensitive to ~~wheat, wheat kernels, wheat germ, and cracked wheat.~~

6. *Supplements*: Talk to your doctor about taking multivitamin and mineral supplements. If you are primarily vegetarian, also ask about taking additional vitamin B12 and zinc supplements.

7. *Drink plenty of pure or filtered water* (8 glasses a day are usually recommended). Avoid soft drinks, sugary drinks, and low calorie drinks with artificial sweeteners.

8. *Avoid sugars, artificial sweeteners, and processed carbohydrates*, as well as high-glycemic index carbohydrates such as sugar, white flour,

muffins, doughnuts, pastries, cakes, pies, sugary commercial breakfast cereals, honey, syrup, white breads and bagels, most crackers, white rice, cookies, chips, and jams.

9. *Avoid foods containing transfats* including margarine, fried foods, vegetable shortening, hydrogenated vegetable oils, commercial pastries and baked food products containing hydrogenated oils (such as white breads, biscuits, cakes, cookies, crackers, doughnuts, muffins, pies and rolls), and most prepared snacks, mixes, and convenience foods.

10. *Avoid red and processed meats and raw eggs*. Also avoid raw fish if you have an impaired health defense system.[52]

Try to focus on eating nutritious foods such as those mentioned in Tips 1 though 5 above as well as the foods listed in Chapter 5 under *What Foods to Focus On*.   It is important to get a healthy dose of vitamins, minerals, antioxidants, essential fatty acids, protein, and other nutrients every day.

2.5. A TEN-MINUTE MAXIMIZED WORKOUT

Thoughts from Isabelle... Me again! Before I began The Ten-Minute Workout, I had not been exercising at all and was a bit skeptical that it would really make a difference. To my surprise, I found that the exercise along with The 3:00 PM Secret lifestyle made dramatic changes to my body. I discovered that I really do have biceps and hipbones! I listened to the frustrations of other people, such as my friend, Jane, who joined a gym so she could exercise an hour a day, but rarely had the time to go.

My exercise was a convenient 10-minute detour from my morning primping routine using an inexpensive weight bench and some hand and ankle weights. It was quick, easy, and effective. Today, I still do the 10-minute workout, but now that I have become strong, I've added other enjoyable physical activities including hiking, mountain climbing, biking,

---

[52] www.cfsan.fda.gov/~ear/FLRECSAF.htm

skiing, running, basketball, martial arts, and yoga. I am stronger and healthier than I thought possible. I never get sick and all the health problems I used to have are distant memories. By strengthening my body, I also made it healthier.

And you know what? Being able to do hard physical activities makes me feel so empowered! This feeling of strength and empowerment transfers over into all aspects of my life. Once you become slim and strong, you never know what you will be inspired to do! Life is an adventure filled with twists, turns, and wonderful surprises. A strong, lithe body will give you the ability and confidence to blaze all kinds of new trails!

Still not convinced exercise is powerful? Here are a few reasons to consider! Exercise will:

(1) Improve your memory and cognitive ability;

(2) Improve your cardiovascular system;

(3) Improve your posture;

(4) Reduce your risk of falling and the resulting fractured or broken bones;

(5) Increase your energy, strength, endurance, balance, flexibility, and muscle tone;

(6) Help ward off osteoporosis by maintaining your bone density;

(7) Relieve depression;

(8) Raise your self-esteem;

(9) Reduce your risk of cardiovascular disease, stroke, diabetes, cancer, and many other diseases;

(10) Improve your sleep;

(11) Increase the blood vessels in and the blood supply to your brain, enabling you to think better;

(12) Increase levels of the chemicals and growth factors in your brain that are involved in motor function, cognition, reasoning, thinking, and learning, and that prevent the connections between nerve cells from breaking down and help them grow back;

(13) Reduce your risk of Alzheimer's disease; and

(14) Reduce age-related disability characterized by generalized weakness, impaired mobility, poor balance, poor endurance, and loss of muscle

strength, which dramatically affect your chances of living an independent life as you age.

Seems pretty convincing to me!

And don't say you're too old. The good news is that, according to researchers, age-related muscle loss can be reversed at *any* age using strength-training exercise. Strength training not only increases muscle mass and strength, but also increases bone density, restores good balance, enhances sleep, and helps people to stay vital and independent as they age. Did you know that loss of muscle strength is a major determinant of whether you will live an independent life as you age? Falls contribute to 40% of admissions to nursing homes. People who refuse to exercise lose strength and balance, and are therefore inadvertently choosing to live in a rest home rather than remaining free and independent. If you want to remain strong and independent throughout your life, *the prevention of frailty that comes with age can only be achieved by **exercise**!*

Most people know that exercise is protective against cardiovascular disease, but did you know that your brain is enhanced through exercise? Evidence is accumulating that exercise has profound benefits for brain function. Physical activity improves learning and memory, and an active lifestyle can prevent or delay loss of cognitive function with aging or neurodegenerative disease.[53] Exercise increases the vasculature and blood supply in the brain and also raises levels of certain chemicals and growth factors.[54] These chemicals that are released from nerve cells during exercise help nerve cells resist illness and injury, prompt them to grow and multiply, and strengthen connections between nerve cells. Not only do these chemicals promote learning and memory, but are believed to help the brain resist Alzheimer's and Parkinson's diseases. Exercise has also been shown to have positive effects at the chromosomal level.[55] A study of monkeys showed running protected neurons in their brains from damage.[56]

I could go on and on about the enormous benefits of exercise. It is protective against cardiovascular disease, dementia, and Alzheimer's disease.

---

[53] Trends in Neurosciences v.32 No.5, p.283-90, May 2009

[54] The Journal of Neuroscience v.20, No.8, p.2926, 4//15/00

[55] Archives of Internal Medicine v.168, No.2, p.154-158, 1/28/08; Science News, v.173, No.5, p.69, 2/2/08

[56] Science News v.176, No.11, p. 8, 11/21/09

Compounding the benefits even further, the Cancer *Report* discussed earlier in this chapter said exercise is protective against a number of cancers. Regular exercise increases lifespan, wards off diseases, and makes you strong and beautiful. Please exercise!

* * * * * * * * * * * * * * * * * * *

FIRST MALE MUSING ON EXERCISE

If you are not giving yourself enough regular physical exercise, do you know **why**? What is really stopping you from building effective exercise into your daily routine? Maybe you think you just don't have time. What would it take for you to **want** to exercise regularly?

Appealing to the intellect won't be enough. You already **know** good muscle tone will help your posture, balance, energy level, and strength. You already **know** toned muscles burn more calories even while you're resting or asleep, helping you keep slim. You already **know** a strong cardiovascular system increases your stamina and longevity. If it were only a matter of knowing the facts, there would be **no** problem. You'd already be in shape! Wouldn't you be happier if you looked and felt better? Wouldn't the pride of a good physique add to your feeling of self-worth? Wouldn't you like yourself more if you commanded enough self-control to get the exercise you need?

So what will it take to at least get you started? What if the first step is quick, easy, convenient, painless, and inexpensive, and yet effective in moving you toward better physical condition? When she designed the 10-minute workouts, Debra had in mind people who were not exercising regularly, didn't think exercise was particularly enjoyable, and were not known for their discipline and self-control. Sound familiar?

She believes if you begin short, easy, convenient daily exercises, within several weeks you will make a habit of it. You will begin to look and feel stronger and will like the results. The better muscle tone will contribute to weight loss by burning more calories even while you rest, and you will soon find yourself quite a ways down the path toward the body you desire. It may seem like a long journey when standing at the starting line, but incremental daily progress through 10-minutes of regular convenient exercise is not an arduous journey, just part of a daily routine, like brushing your teeth.

Once daily exercise becomes a habit for you, you can customize your activities to your particular circumstances and preferences. But to start, just try the 10-minute workout for 10 days. If you like the result, go for 10 more days, and then 10 more. Yes, you can do this!

* * * * * * * * * * * * * * * * * * *

Why Ten Minutes?

Good question since everyone says you need more! In fact, I am a strong advocate of doing nearly daily vigorous exercise for thirty minutes punctuated with regular (weekly) sustained exercise or activity such as an all-day mountain climb. Such activity keeps your cardiovascular system healthy and strengthens your muscles, organs, and physiological systems – not to mention the tremendous psychological benefits. Moreover, I believe combining this type of exercise schedule with an elimination of negative psychological stress can have dramatically positive health benefits. Nevertheless, telling a person who is not accustomed to exercise to immediately adopt a schedule such as this is not practical.

My hope is that a commitment to ten minutes of daily exercise is a good compromise and a good beginning, and may result in more total exercise over time and an appreciation of the transforming impact of vigorous physical activity in your life. If you begin with the Ten-Minute Workout and start to see benefits, you may find new, challenging physical activities within your reach and realize they can be fun, enormously rewarding, and empowering. After you integrate the Ten-Minute Workout into your life, you can increase your workout time or add cycling, swimming, jogging, hiking, tennis, or other enjoyable sports or athletic activities.

If you are already doing thirty to sixty minutes of exercise or going to a gym every day – great! Keep it up! Just make sure you are getting a total-body, strength-training workout along with any aerobics you may be doing.

Muscles Build Strength and Independence

The *10-minute Workout* is centered around weight training. Weight training, also referred to as strength training, resistance training, or weight-bearing exercise, involves lifting, moving, pulling, or pushing against resistance or weight. Weight training will cause you to replace fat tissue with muscle tissue, which will increase your body's metabolism twenty-four hours a day. Increasing muscle tissue will allow you to burn more calories even while you are not exercising because muscle is active tissue, which burns more calories than fat tissue. Weight-bearing exercise will help you ward off osteoporosis by maintaining and restoring bone density, and it will push back the deleterious effects of aging that make you frail and weak. It will improve your balance, endurance, strength, and posture, and make you feel more empowered, attractive, and self-confident. Weight lifting will not only give you a stronger, healthier body, but will enable you to redistribute your weight for a more balanced physique. Weight training is a way for someone who is obese to manage exercise without the pounding of jogging or aerobics.

According to researchers, as humans age beyond 40, approximately one-third to one-half of a pound of muscle is lost each year and replaced by fat. This contributes to a loss of about one to two percent of strength each year.[57] As muscles weaken and movement becomes more difficult, people eventually become more sedentary and dependent. This apparent dismal inevitability of our aging bodies can be slowed and reversed by strength training! Exercise will keep both your body and mind strong, healthy and independent as you age.

Are you averse to weightlifting?

You can still do the daily workout using resistance-providing aerobic exercise equipment for ten to twenty minutes. Examples of resistance-providing aerobic exercise equipment include a Nordic Trac, a rowing machine, an elliptical, a stair climber, a stepper, an exercise bike, or an inclined treadmill. Another great fill-in exercise is repeatedly climbing up and down a set of stairs. (Set a radio nearby or do it with a friend since it is a bit repetitive, but it's a great workout. Also, use the handrail and watch your step!)

---

[57] Miriam Nelson, Ph.D. Tufts University, www.strongwomen.com

Aerobic Exercise

You may want to engage in aerobic exercise along with weight training. Vigorous aerobic exercise and activities are extremely beneficial! After I built up my strength and health with the *Ten-Minute Workout*, I added running, mountain hiking, cross-country skiing, and biking to my regular activities. I am a strong believer that regular, vigorous exercise is crucial to good physical and mental health. Not only does aerobic exercise do wonders for your cardiovascular system, but it has been shown to ease mild or moderate depression nearly as well as a commonly-prescribed antidepressant medication.[58]

If you currently do an aerobic-type of exercise you can add weight training a few days per week in order to create a body with balanced muscle mass and strength. You may also substitute two or three of the ten-minute weight training workouts with *vigorous aerobic exercise* each week. A possible schedule could be doing the ten-minute weight-training workout three days per week and doing a run or bike ride the alternate three days of the week. You can rest on day seven.

Make the Ten-Minute Workout Convenient!

Do you have a place in your home that is very visible and hard to avoid? That is where you should place your weights (and bench or other equipment). It may be in your living room, bedroom, family room, etc. If you want to listen to the radio and look out a window during your workout, then put your equipment nearby. Keep a pair of athletic shoes next to your weights so you can quickly pull them on as you begin your daily workout. Also, wear anything you are comfortable in: a tee-shirt, shorts, stretch pants, night shirt, etc. You should also view yourself in a mirror to check your form (and results).

Equipment and Weights

The only equipment *required* for *The 10-Day Dream Diet* exercise routines in this book is a pair of *dumbbell weights*. There are *alternatives* to some exercises as well as *additional exercises* listed in Appendix 3, which use a

---

[58] Psychosomatic Medicine September 2007; Science News, v.172, No.15, p.237, 10/13/07

standard *weight bench* and *ankle weights*. But to begin with, and especially if you are new to weight lifting, you can just do the primary exercises described for the ten days, which only use dumbbell weights.

Dumbbells are small weights you hold in each hand. If you are new to weight lifting, you will begin with a set of low-weight dumbbells, such as 3 to 8 pounds depending on your strength. You should be able to lift the dumbbells over your head with some effort, but without straining. As you continue to work out, you will want heavier dumbbells, maybe 5 to 10 pounds or more. You can also purchase adjustable dumbbells.

If you decide to do the Hamstring Curls and Quadriceps Extensions described in Appendix 3 as extra exercises, you will need *ankle weights*. Ankle weights are strapped around each ankle and usually range from 1 to 20 pounds. You can begin with a set of lighter ankle weights, such as 3 to 5 pounds, depending on your strength. Adjustable ankle weights are also available.

Breathing

When a body builder is lifting a heavy weight, she breathes out during the lifting phase and in during the lowering phase. When doing this workout, however, you will be moving quickly and smoothly through an exercise faster than your natural rhythm of breathing, so breathe normally. It is very important to keep breathing and not to hold your breath, which you may find yourself doing inadvertently.

Stretching

Every day you need to stretch. It is best to stretch just after your workout, but you can do it anytime during the day or evening. Here are three stretches you should do every day:

1. Sit on the floor with your legs straight in front of you. While keeping your legs and back straight, lean forward and reach for and hold onto (if you can) your toes. Hold it for a count of 100.

2. Sit on the floor and spread your legs to the sides as far as possible. While keeping your legs and back straight, reach toward your right foot, and hold

your toes (if you can) for a count of 100. Then reach for your left foot and hold it for a count of 100.

3. Stretch your calves one at a time. Stand up with the ball of one foot resting on a thick book and the heel of that same foot on the floor. Hold it for the count of 100. Switch to the other leg and do the same.

The Workout

If you read *The 3:00 PM Secret: Live Slim and Strong Live Your Dreams*, you will notice the exercises in this book look familiar. I did not want to overwhelm those who have not lifted weights before with too many different exercises, so *The 10 Day Dream Diet* plan in this book includes five standard upper-body exercises and five (or six) standard lower-body exercises. Additional exercises are included in Appendix 3 so they can be used if you repeat *The 10 Day Dream Diet* and want to expand your exercise. The upper-body and lower-body exercises should be done on alternate days for the ten-day period and are:

UPPER-BODY EXERCISES FOR DAYS 1, 3, 5, 7, and 9:
Shoulders-SIDE RAISE; Biceps-CURL;
Back-BENT LIFT; Triceps-PUSHBACK;
Chest-PUSHUPS or BENCH PRESS (if you have a bench).

LOWER-BODY EXERCISES FOR DAYS 2, 4, 6, 8, and 10:
Calves-STANDING STRAIGHT-TOE RAISE;
Quadriceps/Glut-SQUAT; Hamstring-LUNGE;
Abdominal-LEG LOWERING; Abdominal-CRUNCH;
Abdominal-ALTERNATE TWIST (Extra).

If you are short of time or tired on any particular day, still do the workout – just do fewer repetitions of each exercise. You want to get into the habit of doing a workout every day even if it is only minutes.

When you begin doing new exercises, you can expect that the muscles you work one day may be somewhat sore the next day. Soreness means you are developing your muscles. Do not, however, push yourself beyond your limit until you experience pain or injure yourself. An injury will set you back and slow your progress. Challenge yourself when you work out, but don't push until the muscles you are working experience pain.

Note: If you are new to weight training, you may want to schedule an appointment with a professional trainer or expert to help you begin your ten-minute workout plan. Talk to your doctor before starting any exercise program, especially if you have health problems or have not exercised for a long time.

2.6. SLEEP

Don't turn to food for the energy you should be getting from sleep.

THOUGHTS ON SLEEP…
When you lack it, life seems arduous and murky.
With a slight shortage, you cope, survive, and manage.
With a full dose, you lightly dance through daily tasks with
optimism, buoyancy, and jubilance.
When trials come, it provides clarity for prudent decisions and actions.
Sleep is crucial for health, happiness, and optimism.

Rest in the Lord, and wait patiently for him… Psalms 37:7
It is vain for you to rise up early, to sit up late, to eat the bread of sorrows:
for so He giveth his beloved sleep. Psalms 127:2

Thoughts from Isabelle… *I remember explaining to my friend, Ellen, that I don't need an afternoon pick-me-up snack because I get eight hours of sleep at night. The reason I get enough sleep is I don't do the fix/eat/cleanup dinner ritual and then sit in front of the boob tube at night wasting my life. I have learned to spend my evenings living – not watching.*

Do you think sleep is a waste of time? I used to. But now I realize that by giving myself adequate sleep, I am healthier and my awake-time is happier and more productive. I think more clearly, feel more buoyant, and get more accomplished. If you are trying to lose weight, sleep problems can exacerbate weight problems. When we do not get adequate and healthy sleep, we become tired and drag ourselves around. This lethargic condition causes us to burn fewer calories. When we are sleep deprived, we are also less likely to exercise. Further, when we are tired and need energy, we eat "just to get through the day", and are more likely to choose sugary, unhealthy foods. Eating for the energy you should be getting from sleep is a mistake and can sabotage your efforts to lose weight.

Researchers have been examining the link between sleep and excess body weight. Some researchers believe this connection may be due to sleep's effect on the blood levels of hunger and satiety hormones that affect eating behavior.[59] Studies have found that sleep-deprived adults produced more hunger-promoting gherelin and less hunger-suppressing leptin, thereby encouraging food intake. They exhibited an increase in hunger and appetite, which encouraged excess eating and made weight loss difficult. It was found that sleep duration is also an important regulator of metabolism.[60] Sleeping less than 7 to 8 hours at night has been linked to both obesity and diabetes. People who sleep less also produce markedly elevated amounts of insulin, which reflects a state of insulin resistance – a common predictor of diabetes.[61] Other studies suggest a direct connection between inadequate sleep and insulin resistance, diabetes, cardiovascular disease, low-grade inflammation, and hormonal changes that promote weight gain.[62] Even one night of short sleep increases levels of inflammatory chemicals and hunger-promoting hormones in the blood. Getting too little sleep increases your chances of losing their health and speeding up deaths arrival either by disease or accident. Sleeping seven to eight hours per night decreases your risk of obesity, diabetes, heart disease, and other illnesses.[63] There is even a link between inadequate sleep and Alzheimer's disease.[64] Inadequate sleep is associated with accumulating levels of the Beta-amyloid deposits in the brain, which is thought to be the initiating event in the development of Alzheimer's disease.[65]

---

[59] Science News v.167, No.14 Pg.216, 5/2/05

[60] Annuals of Internal Medicine; v.141, No.11, p.846-850, 12/7/04; Science News, v.169, No.13, p.195, 4/1/06

[61] Science News, v.169, No.13, p.195, 4/1/06

[62] Science News v.162 No.10, p.152-154, 9/7/02; Science News v.174, No.8, p.14, 10/11/09; Science News v.175, No.1, p.5-6, 1/3/09

[63] Science News v.176, No.9, Pg.28-32, 10/24/09

[64] Science News v.176, No.9, p.11, 10/24/09

[65] Science v.326, p.1005-1007, 11/13/09

When we are asleep, biochemical processes occur that are critical to the healthy functioning of our bodies. During sleep, sugars are stored, the body temperature decreases which conserves energy, and various hormones and chemicals (prolactin, cortisol, and growth hormone) are released into the bloodstream. The immune system is boosted during sleep, and there are increased levels of immune system chemicals such as interleukin-1 and tumor necrosis factor (which is a killer of cancer cells) in the blood.[66]

A top priority should be soundly sleeping 7 to 8 hours every night.

* * * * * * * * * * * * * * * * * *

MALE MUSING ON SLEEP

Perhaps you have learned through experience how sleep deprivation degrades a person's perspective and ability to cope with the demands of life. Extensive sleep deprivation results in disintegration of personality and a form of insanity. So, if you only burn your candle at both ends to a limited degree, you're only a little crazy and warped!

As a habitual high-energy high-achiever, I once took pride in surviving on only five or six hours of sleep. My "late to bed – early to rise" lifestyle began in high school with early classes and homework performed after evening athletic practices. I presumed that lesser beings who coddled themselves with eight or more hours of sleep were lazy, self-indulgent underachievers, destined to be unconscious during many of life's best moments.

Over the years I proudly wore emblems of my successful wakefulness, including red baggy eyes, catnaps during meetings, and even a near-fatal accident after driving all night and falling asleep at the wheel while listening to a book-on-tape.

As you may suspect, none of these promptings motivated me to alter my habits. I did not change until I had a few months between job assignments on an extended honeymoon with an unrepentant sleeper. Now Debra is not a lazy, self-indulgent underachiever, but a very hard-working and focused achiever. She also does not fall asleep in the middle of the day and constantly looks bright-eyed.

---

[66] The Promise of Sleep, William C. Dement, M.D., Ph.D. , Delacorte Press 1999 p.258,266,268

Without deliberately embarking on an experiment, I began to average almost eight hours of sleep per night. My alarm clock was usually a rowdy poodle, later known as "GlacierDog", except for days when he was preempted by an errant woodpecker.

My sample size of one is inadequate and the results predictable, but I will report them anyway. The red baggy-eye phenomenon disappeared. I remained alert all day long without stimulants except for the excitement of life. I coped better with significant uncertainty and stress and maintained a sunnier disposition. My waking hours were slightly fewer but of higher quality. I had time and energy to complete everything that needed doing and more.

The body and mind both use the hours of sleep to repair the ravages of the day and prepare for the next. If you curtail these important natural processes, you will not only look and feel a bit like a zombie, but over the long run you will damage your health.

Think of your efforts to obtain good nutrition and exercise as slowing the burn rate on your candle of life. If extending the life of your candle is important to you, why would you deliberately burn your candle on the other end by being sleep-deprived?

Sleep really feels good and is at least as important as all your nutritional supplements or carefully selected organic foods. And sleep is free! Why feel guilty about it? If you need to excuse yourself early from an event to go home to bed, just say you need to go home to work on an important reconstruction and restoration project. Everyone will be impressed by your industriousness! Then delegate those tasks to the little men inside your body and mind that do the nocturnal repair work while you enjoy a good dream. What's not to like about that?

If you're feeling a little frayed at the edges, remember MacBeth's observation that sleep "knits up the raveled sleeve of care."

* * * * * * * * * * * * * * * * * * *

PART II

Chapter 3

The 10-Day Dream Diet

Chapter 4

Lifestyle Secrets and Inspirations from Alaska to the World

Chapter 5

What's Next?

Chapter 3

The 10-Day Dream Diet

The following pages lay out the *10-Day Dream Diet.* Here is a summary of what you will be doing:

Eat breakfast, lunch, and a 2:30 snack – Follow the suggested menus in this chapter. You may make substitutions of similar foods if necessary.

Do at least 10-minutes of exercise – Follow the provided exercises, choose a similar alternative, or expand to both strength training and aerobic exercise.

Answer your *dream* question of the day – Read the daily "Words for Thought" and answer your daily "Dream Question".

If necessary, have a glass of warm milk, soymilk, or juice in the evening

Sleep 7 to 8 hours each night.

There is a shopping list in Appendix 6 to assist you with buying foods necessary for the menus. Read through the menus and refine the shopping list according to your preferences before you begin.

If you begin the *10-Day Dream Diet* and it gets interrupted, do not get frustrated and give up – just begin again. My hope is that you will have such success with *The 3:00 PM Secret* lifestyle you will adopt it as a permanent practice – and never be plagued by weight issues again! If this is the case, then adopting it through the *10-Day Dream Diet* will feel like an ongoing process and interruptions will be just that – interruptions – not permanent deterrents. If you practice *The 3:00 PM Secret*, I believe you will lose your desire to have a meal at night, so it will not feel like a restriction but a liberating choice you will never want to give up as a normal practice. You will be slim, strong, and in control of yourself, and you will have the confidence to live your dream life.

When you begin not eating a meal at night, you will be fighting against a tradition of "dinner eating" rather than an actual physical need for food. It takes a while to get used to not eating a meal at night, but once you get past the first weeks or months, you will feel liberated and will be happy with the effect on your body and life. One of the benefits of the 3:00 PM lifestyle is that by not eating a meal at night when you really do not need the food for nutrition, your brain learns to associate eating with a biological need rather than comfort, self-nurture, or habit. Eventually you will find you have lost your desire to eat for the wrong reasons and will be liberated and in control of your body and life.

The 3:00 PM Secret 10 Day Dream Diet is NOT about the food. Food is for nourishment not for satisfying emotional needs, comfort, habit-eating, or stuffing down your disappointments. Focus on your "*Dream*" question each day. *The 3:00 PM Secret* lifestyle is about living your dream life and finding and fulfilling your purposes.

* * * * * * * * * * * * * * * * * * *

MALE MUSING ON RECIPES

For a person with a weight-control problem, it is dangerous to spend too much time in or around food. We've all heard about the "see food" diet! If you don't want to find yourself drinking, cowboy, don't hitch your horse in front of the saloon. Yet so many "diet" books spend endless pages on elaborate recipes that require hours of food shopping and preparation when food is the **last** thing the reader should be contemplating. So why offer menus in this book?

Well, these meal suggestions illustrate that your daily food events can be nutritious, low in calories, tasty, simple, quick, and free of toxins and questionable additives. Unless your dream is to be a chef, your future does not lie in a kitchen! Don't just keep a physical distance from the refrigerator and cupboard, keep a mental distance too. These simple meals are designed to give you the nutrition your body needs while downplaying food as a central event in your life.

When I began my change a few years ago from a mediocre bachelor diet toward the healthy organic prescriptions of the author of *The 3:00 PM Secret*, I consulted several excellent healthy, organic, vegetarian cookbooks she had on hand. We selected the ones that sounded best and made shopping lists of the necessary ingredients. I looked forward to preparing exciting new healthy recipes. Life would be wonderful.

The shopping trip took **forever**. The exciting new recipes had long lists of ingredients, many difficult or impossible to find. We did the best we could and returned home tired but not entirely discouraged. It was too late for elaborate cooking so we made do with whatever food was in the refrigerator, throwing together an unnamed random salad. We'd make cooking history the next day.

The next day we started early and followed an elaborate recipe as closely as possible. It felt like a chemistry experiment, and we didn't dare deviate in case something might explode or at least not turn out perfect. After over an hour of collaboration and sneaking of snacks to quell our growing hunger, we sat down to a very nice though overly-spicy concoction. After the brief meal we faced another project – cleaning up and putting away after our culinary opus. The entire undertaking took well over two hours (not including the shopping expedition).

It then dawned on me that the meal process we had just been through resulted in the consumption of a very nicely prepared dish that was not as nutritious or tasty as the miscellaneous salad we had thrown together in less than 10 minutes the day before. I also realized that in following the recipe I felt confined and frustrated, as if I was under the authority of the person behind the formula. By comparison, putting together a quick meal from the available ingredients tapped our creativity and sense of adventure.

As a result of this and similar experiences, our practical and fun approach to meals has evolved into an efficient and enjoyable experience. Every week or two we purchase a collection of vegetables, greens, fruits, nut butters, breads, juices, cereals, yogurt, tofu, and other primarily unprocessed, organic foods. We mix, stir fry, steam, or otherwise combine them as the spirit moves us, making enough for two or three days of meals. Then we exit the kitchen, put food out of our minds, and pursue whatever fun, interesting, or profitable activity is next on our agenda.

Ironically, one of those activities turns out to be sharing some of our favorite ad hoc meal ideas with you. But don't feel imprisoned or dictated to by these prescriptions – they are only suggestions to help you get started with quick, simple, and nutritious meals. You can find enjoyment in making up your own quick and easy new combinations of good basic foods that will keep you healthy and mostly *out of the kitchen*. You can even make up names for your creations. If you call it "Aunt Tillie's Spinach Delight" your guests won't realize that you made it all up from what was on hand that morning!

* * * * * * * * * * * * * * * * * * *

Eating journal: An Eating Journal can be beneficial if you are not losing weight fast enough and cannot figure out why. It also adds a psychological barrier to eating what you know you should not, if you have to tattle on yourself by writing it down. If you are dropping pounds at a reasonable rate, feel "in control", and it seems like a hassle, then don't bother.

A few notes before getting started

It is OK to vary the order of the menu days such as swapping Day 1's menu with Day 4's menu. Note that lunches on Days 2 and 3, Days 5 and 6, and Days 8 and 9 are prepared on Days 2, 5, and 8, respectively. It is also OK to make like substitutions such as lettuce for spinach, any healthy hot cereal for oatmeal, or goat's milk for milk or soymilk. Also, proteins such as tempeh, tofu, salmon, tuna, organic egg, etc., are interchangeable. Along with the suggested meals, I also recommend consuming flaxseed oil, flaxseed oil supplements, or fish oil supplements daily.

The portions given in the menus are for one person. They are *approximate* and will depend on your height, gender, and activity level. For example, if you are a six-foot man, you will want to increase the portions by 50% to 100%. Conversely, if you are a 5 foot 2 inch woman and you are trying to lose that "last ten pounds", you may need to slightly lighten up. The best approach is to follow your weight loss and modify how much you eat according to how you are losing. This is where an Eating Journal would come in handy.

It is important that you discuss this new eating style with your doctor (especially if you have or are prone to diabetes) and verify that he or she confirms that not eating a meal (except perhaps a glass of juice, soymilk, etc., or a piece of fruit) between 3:00 p.m. and 6:00 p.m. (or when you get up) the next morning is acceptable for you. Also, if you have a special diet indicated by your doctor and your doctor gives you permission to not eat a meal after 3:00 p.m. for 10 days, then eat your last meal before 3:00 p.m.

DAY 1

Record starting weight_____lbs.

Suggested menu – Portions are for one person. Double, triple, etc., for more people. Adjust portions according to height and body type: a muscular six-foot man may increase portions by 50% to 100%, and a small-boned, short woman may need to slightly decrease portions. Weigh yourself to see that you are losing weight at a reasonable rate and adjust accordingly.

Breakfast: Granola, Yogurt, and Fruit

- ½ to 1 cup granola with rice milk (or other milk)
- 1 cup plain organic yogurt mixed with 1 cup strawberries or other fruit
- Grapefruit or unsweetened juice
- Herbal or green tea or coffee

Lunch: Open-Faced Tuna Melt (or Sandwich)

- Tuna (or salmon) melt – mix:
  - ½ cup or small can of tuna or salmon,
  - 1-2 tablespoons organic plain yogurt,
  - 2 tablespoons organic cottage cheese or 1 ounce hard cheese,
  - Dill weed, ginger, and turmeric.
  - Load onto 2 slices of toast & broil in toaster oven or broiler 4-5 min.
  - Alternatively, make into a tuna sandwich.
  - You may substitute hard-boiled egg, tofu, or tempeh for fish.
- Water and/or herbal tea

2:30 PM Snack:

- 1 piece fruit and drink plenty of water

Evening: (If necessary)

- 1 cup juice, soymilk, or warm milk/soymilk with cinnamon and nutmeg

Tip: The easiest place to exercise self-control over what you eat is at your front door. If you don't want to eat it, **keep it out of your house**.

DAY 1: 10-MINUTE WORKOUT

Remember to breathe.

Shoulders--SIDE RAISE (Repeat 30 times)

Start/Finish position: Stand with feet shoulder-width apart, abdominal muscles tightened, and knees unlocked. Hold dumbbells down in front of your thighs with palms facing inward.

While keeping elbows slightly bent, extend and raise dumbbells out from your sides in arc-movements until they are level with your shoulders and your palms are facing down, which is the Midpoint position. Pause briefly. While keeping arms nearly straight and palms facing down, lower dumbbells back down in arc-movements to the Start/Finish position.

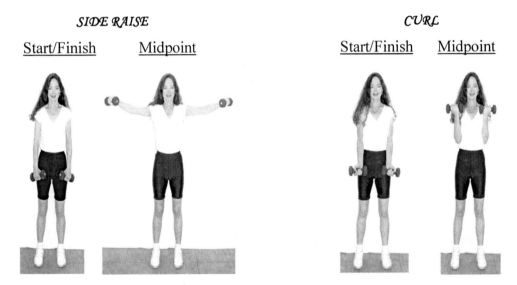

SIDE RAISE   CURL

Start/Finish   Midpoint   Start/Finish   Midpoint

Biceps--CURL (Repeat 30-40 times)

Start/Finish position: Stand with feet shoulder-width apart, abdominal muscles tightened, and knees unlocked. Hold dumbbells down close to your sides and slightly in front of your thighs with palms facing forward.

Keeping your upper arms stationary with elbows against waist, bend elbows, and raise dumbbells up to your shoulders in an arc-motion so that palms are facing your shoulders in the Midpoint position. Pause briefly. Lower dumbbells back down in an arc-motion to Start/Finish position.

Back--BENT LIFT (Repeat 40 times)

Start/Finish position: Stand with feet shoulder-width apart. Bend forward at waist, look straight ahead, and keep knees slightly bent. Your spine should be straight and shoulders should not be rounded. Hold dumbbells straight down with palms facing back toward your legs.

Keeping palms facing back, lift dumbbells, drawing your elbows up toward the ceiling in a rowing motion until the dumbbells are outside of and slightly lower than your shoulders to the Midpoint position. Squeeze shoulder blades together and pause briefly. Keeping palms facing back, lower dumbbells back down to Start/Finish position.

BENT LIFT		PUSHBACK	
Start/Finish	Midpoint	Start/Finish	Midpoint

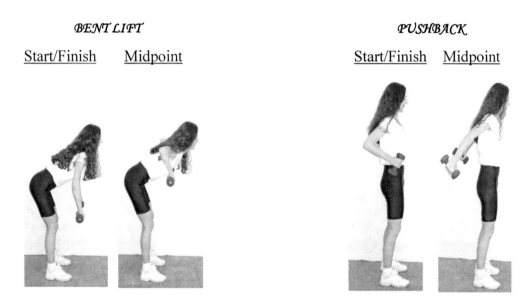

Triceps--PUSHBACK (Repeat 30-40 times)

Start/Finish position: Stand with knees slightly bent. Look ahead and down slightly. Hold dumbbells close to your sides near your hips with palms facing inward and your upper arms and elbows pointing back.

While keeping your palms facing each other, your upper arms steady, and elbows pointing back, extend dumbbells back in arc-movements to the Midpoint position. Pause briefly. Move dumbbells down and forward in arc-movements back to the Start/Finish position.

Chest--PUSH-UP *(Repeat 20 to 40 times)*

Start/Finish position: Lie on your stomach, slightly lifting your body off the floor using your hands and toes (for boy pushup) or using hands and knees (for girl pushup). Do "girl" pushups if you are just beginning.

Push yourself up, keeping back straight, until your elbows are straight to the Midpoint position. Pause briefly. Lower yourself back down to Start/Finish position.

Start/Finish   Midpoint

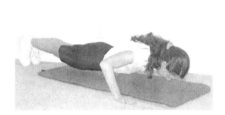 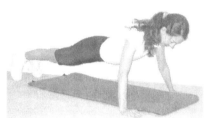

Alternate for Push-up if you have a weight bench:

Chest--BENCH PRESS *(Repeat 40 times)*

Start/Finish position: Lie on your back on a bench. Hold dumbbells just above your shoulders with palms facing up and elbows pointing down.

Press dumbbells straight up over your chest to the Midpoint position and continue to press. Pause briefly. Lower dumbbells to Start/Finish position.

Start/Finish   Midpoint

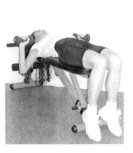 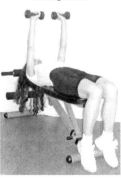

ANSWER YOUR DREAM QUESTION:

1. *If you had twenty million dollars in the bank and never needed to work again, how would you spend your time for the rest of your life?*

_____

_____

_____

_____

_____

_____

_____

_____

_____

_____

_____

_____

_____

_____

WORDS FOR THOUGHT

I will instruct thee and teach thee in the way which thou shalt go: I will guide thee with mine eye. Psalm 32:8.

There hath no temptation taken you but such as is common to man: but God is faithful, who will not suffer you to be tempted above that ye are able; but will with the temptation also make a way to escape, that ye may be able to bear it. 1 Corinthians 10:13.

SLEEP 7 TO 8 HOURS

DAY 2

Record your weight_____lbs.

Suggested menu – Portions are for one person. Double, triple, etc., for more people. Adjust portions according to height and body type. Weigh yourself to see that you are losing weight at a reasonable rate and adjust accordingly.

Breakfast: Oatmeal, Yogurt, and Fruit

- *1 cup cooked oatmeal with 5 walnut or pecan halves and cinnamon*
- *1 cup plain organic yogurt mixed with 1 cup blueberries or other fruit*
- *Vegetable juice or unsweetened fruit juice*
- *Herbal or green tea or coffee*

Lunch: Spinach and Avocado Salad
Makes two servings *for Day 2 and Day 3 Lunches - *eat half* on each day.*
(This will free you from preparing a Day 3 lunch.)

- *Spinach salad with:*
    4 cups spinach,
    1 avocado,
    1 cup cooked beans, rice, fish, or tempeh,
    2 tablespoons sesame seeds,
    2 tablespoons flaxseed oil or olive oil,
    Turmeric, ginger, or favorite spices, lemon juice.
- *Water or herbal tea*

2:30 PM Snack:

- *1 piece of fruit and drink plenty of water*

Evening: *(If necessary)*

- *1 cup juice, soymilk, or warm milk/soymilk with cinnamon and nutmeg*

Tip: Are there certain foods you always seem to overeat? Don't let these "trigger foods" into your house.

DAY 2: 10-MINUTE WORKOUT
Remember to breathe.

Calves--STRAIGHT-TOE RAISE (Repeat 30-40 times)

Start/Finish position: Stand with legs straight and feet shoulder-width apart. Point feet forward and hold a dumbbell in each hand down at your sides with palms facing inward.

While keeping legs straight, raise up on your toes as far as possible to the Midpoint position. Lower back down until your heels are touching the floor to the Start/Finish position. (Remember to stretch calves after this exercise.)

STRAIGHT-TOE RAISE   LEG LOWERING

Start/Finish   Midpoint   Start/Finish   Midpoint

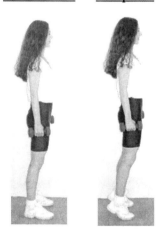
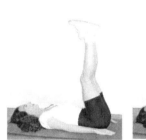
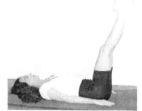

Abdominal--LEG LOWERING (Repeat 30-40 times)

Start/Finish position: Lie on your back on the floor or on a pad with arms down at your sides and hands slightly under your hips. Keeping the middle of your back touching the floor, hold legs up in the air with your feet together and knees slightly bent.

Keeping the middle of your back against the floor, lower legs about 12 inches (or more if able) to the Midpoint position. Pause briefly. Lift legs back up to the Start/Finish position.

Quadriceps/Glut--SQUAT *(Repeat 40 times)*

Start/Finish position: Stand with feet shoulder-width apart. Point feet slightly outward and hold a dumbbell in each hand at your sides with palms facing inward.

While keeping arms down and your back, head, and shoulders straight and nearly upright, bend knees and lower hips until your upper legs are approaching parallel with the floor, as if you are going to sit in a chair, to the Midpoint position. Note: You may actually lower yourself and sit on a chair. Be careful not to lower yourself too far to avoid straining your knees. Raise your body back up to Start/Finish position.

SQUAT	LUNGE
Start/Finish Midpoint	Start/Finish Midpoint

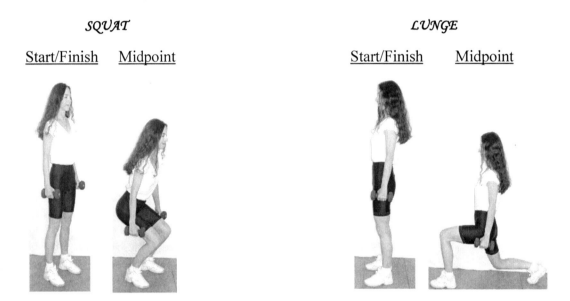

HAMSTRING—LUNGE *(Repeat each leg 40 times)*

Start/Finish position: Stand with feet shoulder-width apart. Point feet forward and hold a dumbbell in each hand at your sides with palms facing in.

While keeping arms down and your back, head, and shoulders straight and upright, step forward with your left foot, bending knees and lowering hips until your right knee is several inches above the floor, or as close to the floor as you are comfortable, to the Midpoint position. The knee of your forward leg should not go past your forward foot. Push with forward leg, raising your body back up and step back to Start/Finish position.

Repeat by stepping forward with right foot and lowering left knee.

ABDOMINAL—CRUNCH (Repeat 40 times)

<u>Start/Finish</u> position: Lie on your back on the floor or a pad with knees shoulder width apart and bent and feet flat on the floor. Keeping your shoulders on the floor, lift your head so that your chin is close to touching your chest (you are looking toward your knees) and your arms are reaching toward your knees.

Keeping your chin to your chest, lift your shoulders up from the floor as your hands reach further between your knees to the <u>Midpoint</u> position. Pause briefly. Lower your shoulders back down to the floor to the <u>Start/Finish</u> position, keeping your chin close to your chest.

<u>Start/Finish</u>   <u>Midpoint</u>

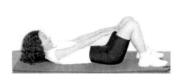 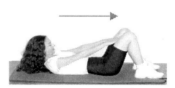

ABDOMINAL--ALTERNATE TWIST (Repeat 40 times)

<u>Start</u> position: Lie on your back on the floor or on a pad. Hold your arms behind your head with fingers just touching your head behind your ears, knees bent and pointing up, and feet flat on the floor.

Point your right leg half way between straight up and the floor and raise your left knee back toward your right shoulder while pointing your right elbow toward your left knee. Your left elbow is on the floor. This is <u>Midpoint</u> position 1.

Switch the positions of your legs while rotating your shoulders so that your left leg is pointing half way between straight up and the floor, your right knee is pointing back toward your left shoulder, and your left elbow is pointing toward your right knee. Your right elbow is on the floor. This is <u>Midpoint</u> position 2. Switch back and forth by rotating shoulders and reversing leg positions to alternate between the two midpoint positions.

<u>Start</u>   <u>Midpoint 1</u>: Right leg out,   <u>Midpoint 2</u>: Left leg out,
                          left knee back,   right knee back,
                       left elbow on floor.   right elbow on floor.

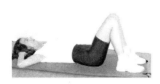 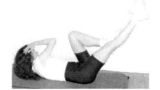 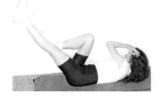

ANSWER YOUR DREAM QUESTION:

2. If you were going to be taken off Earth in 3 years, how would you spend the next 3 years?

_____

_____

_____

_____

_____

_____

_____

_____

_____

_____

_____

_____

_____

_____

WORDS FOR THOUGHT

For yourselves know perfectly that the day of the Lord so cometh as a thief in the night. I Thessalonians 5:2.

Trust in the LORD with all thine heart; and lean not unto thine own understanding. In all thy ways acknowledge him, and he shall direct thy paths. Proverbs 3:5-6.

SLEEP 7 TO 8 HOURS

DAY 3

Record your weight_____lbs.

Suggested menu — Portions are for one person. Double, triple, etc., for more people. Adjust portions according to height and body type. Weigh yourself to see that you are losing weight at a reasonable rate and adjust accordingly.

Breakfast: Cottage Cheese Danish and Fruit

- Toast 2 pieces dense, multigrain bread and spread evenly each with:
    ½ cup organic cottage cheese mixed with cinnamon and nutmeg.
    Broil in toaster oven or broiler for up to 5 minutes.
- 1 cup blueberries or seasonal fruit
- Herbal or green tea, coffee, and/or low-sugar fruit or vegetable juice

Lunch: Spinach and Avocado Salad
Second half of Day 2's Lunch

- Second half of spinach salad from Day 2
- Water or herbal tea

2:30 PM Snack:

- An orange or seasonal fruit and drink plenty of water

Evening: (If necessary)

- 1 cup juice, soymilk, or warm milk/soymilk with cinnamon and nutmeg

Tip: *Manage the need to feed others at night. Prepare a healthy dinner for your children and save your portion in the refrigerator to enjoy the next day for lunch. If possible, shift their dinner slightly earlier.*

DAY 3: 10-MINUTE WORKOUT
(Descriptions on DAY 1)
Repeat each exercise 30-40 times, and remember to breathe.

Biceps—Curl

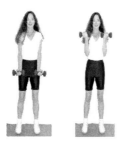

Shoulders--Side Raise

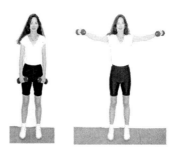

Back--Bent Lift

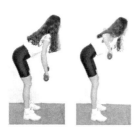

Triceps--Pushback

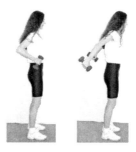

Chest-Push-Ups

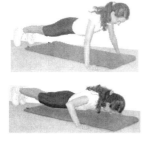

ALTERNATE: Chest-Bench Press

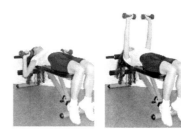

ANSWER YOUR DREAM QUESTION:

3. *You are now 98 years old. What are the 10 things you wish you had done during your life?*

1. _____

2. _____

3. _____

4. _____

5. _____

6. _____

7. _____

8. _____

9. _____

10. _____

WORDS FOR THOUGHT

For which cause we faint not; but though our outward man perish, yet the inward man is renewed day by day. For our light affliction, which is but for a moment, worketh for us a far more exceeding and eternal weight of glory; While we look not at the things which are seen, but at the things which are not seen: for the things which are seen are temporal; but the things which are not seen are eternal. II Corinthians 4:16-18.

Thy word is a lamp unto my feet, and a light unto my path. Psalm 119:105.

SLEEP 7 TO 8 HOURS

DAY 4

Record your weight_____lbs.

Suggested menu – Portions for one person. Double, triple, etc., for more people. Adjust portions according to height and body type. Weigh yourself to see that you are losing weight at a reasonable rate and adjust accordingly.

Breakfast: Smoothie – Toast and Nut butter

- A smoothie made of:
  - 1 cup blueberries, 1 (frozen) banana, rice or soy milk, and 1 cup plain organic yogurt.
- 1 slice whole-grain toast with 1 tablespoon almond butter (or other nut or seed butter)
- Herbal or green tea, coffee, and/or low-sugar fruit or vegetable juice

Lunch: Stuffed Pita Bread

- Pita bread (use regular whole grain bread if you cannot find pita bread) stuffed with:
  - ½ to ¾ cup humus or mashed tofu, tempeh, albacore tuna, or wild salmon mixed with 2 to 3 tablespoons of plain yogurt, ginger, turmeric, and a generous amount of spinach and tomatoes.
- A pear or seasonal fruit
- Water or herbal tea

2:30 PM Snack:

- Carrot and celery sticks and drink plenty of water

Evening: (If necessary)

- 1 cup juice, soymilk, or warm milk/soymilk with cinnamon and nutmeg

Tip: *Have something soothing to drink to take the edge off nighttime hunger.*

DAY 4: 10-MINUTE WORKOUT

(Descriptions on DAY 2)
Repeat each exercise 30-40 times, and remember to breathe.

Calves-Straight-Toe Raise

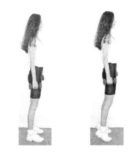

Quadriceps/Glut-Squat

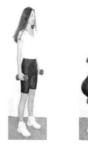

Hamstring-Lunge

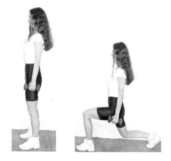

Abdominal-Crunch

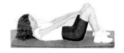

Abdominal-Leg Lowering

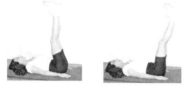

EXTRA EXERCISE:
Abdominal-Alternate Twist

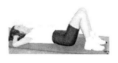

Alternate legs & arms

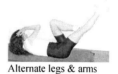

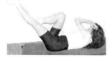

ANSWER YOUR DREAM QUESTION:

4. What do you believe God wants you to do with your life?

_____

_____

_____

_____

_____

_____

_____

_____

_____

_____

_____

_____

_____

_____

_____

WORDS FOR THOUGHT

Abide in me, and I in you. As the branch cannot bear fruit of itself, except it abide in the vine; no more can ye, except ye abide in me. I am the vine, ye are the branches: He that abideth in me, and I in him, the same bringeth forth much fruit: for without me ye can do nothing. If a man abide not in me, he is cast forth as a branch, and is withered; and men gather them, and cast them into the fire, and they are burned. If ye abide in me, and my words abide in you, ye shall ask what ye will, and it shall be done unto you. John 15:4-7.

SLEEP 7 TO 8 HOURS

DAY 5

Record your weight_____lbs.

Suggested menu – Portions are for one person. Double, triple, etc., for more people. Adjust portions according to height and body type. Weigh yourself to see that you are losing weight at a reasonable rate and adjust accordingly.

Breakfast: "Late for Work" Yogurt Nut Butter Blend and Fruit

- Stir 3 tablespoons almond butter (or other nut or seed butter) into
    1 cup organic plain yogurt
- 1 cup or piece of seasonal fruit
- Herbal or green tea, coffee, and/or low-sugar fruit or vegetable juice

Lunch: Stir-Fry (or raw salad) Vegetables
Makes two servings for Day 5 and Day 6 Lunches - eat half

- Stir-Fry about 2 cups vegetables (broccoli, cauliflower, etc.) with
    2 tablespoons olive oil
    Mix in:
        1 cup tofu,
        1 cup chickpeas or beans OR 1 cup cooked wild or brown rice,
        1 small can water chestnuts drained,
        Tamari sauce, turmeric, ginger, cayenne pepper.
    (Optional to just mix up as a salad if no time to stir fry.)
- Water or herbal tea

2:30 PM Snack:

- Vegetable juice, a piece of fruit, and drink plenty of water

Evening: (If necessary)

- 1 cup juice, soymilk, or warm milk/soymilk with cinnamon and nutmeg

Tip: Avoid grocery shopping on an empty stomach and do not sabotage yourself by buying large quantities of your favorite foods. It may seem as if you are saving money by purchasing food in bulk, but you're not saving money or helping yourself when you buy extra food if you end up overeating it.

DAY 5: 10-MINUTE WORKOUT
(Descriptions on DAY 1)
Repeat each exercise 30-40 times, and remember to breathe.

Biceps—Curl

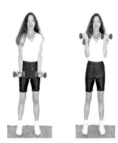

Shoulders--Side Raise

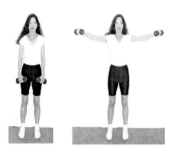

Back--Bent Lift

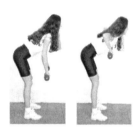

Triceps--Pushback

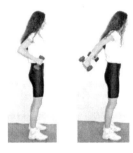

Chest-Push-Ups

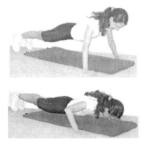

ALTERNATE: Chest-Bench Press

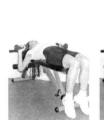
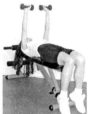

ANSWER YOUR DREAM QUESTION:

5. List 3 or 4 activities you most enjoy doing with your free time. (A benefit of The 3:00 PM Secret is more free time in the evenings.)

_____

_____

_____

_____

_____

_____

_____

_____

_____

_____

_____

_____

_____

_____

_____

WORDS FOR THOUGHT

But seek ye first the kingdom of God, and his righteousness; and all these things shall be added unto you. Matthew 6:33.

Jesus said unto him, Thou shalt love the Lord thy God with all thy heart, and with all thy soul, and with all thy mind. This is the first and great commandment. And the second is like unto it, Thou shalt love thy neighbour as thyself. On these two commandments hang all the law and the prophets. Matthew 22:37-40.

SLEEP 7 TO 8 HOURS

DAY 6

Record your weight____lbs.

Suggested menu – Portions are for one person. Double, triple, etc., for more people. Adjust portions according to height and body type. Weigh yourself to see that you are losing weight at a reasonable rate and adjust accordingly.

Breakfast: Scrambled Eggs (or tofu) and Yogurt and Fruit

- *2 organic eggs (or 1 cup tofu) scrambled with:*
   1 to 2 tablespoons soy or other milk, ¼ cup organic cottage cheese or 1 ounce hard cheese, and ginger and turmeric
- *1 cup plain organic yogurt mixed with 1 cup seasonal fruit*
- *Herbal or green tea, coffee, and/or low-sugar fruit or vegetable juice*

Lunch: Stir-Fry (or raw salad) Vegetables
Second half of Day 5's lunch
(Enjoy not having to prepare a lunch today.)

- *Second half of Stir-Fry vegetables (or salad) from Day 5*
- *Water or herbal tea*

2:30 PM Snack:

- *Apple, pear, or orange and drink plenty of water*

Evening: (If necessary)

- *1 cup juice, soymilk, or warm milk/soymilk with cinnamon and nutmeg*

Tip: Turn off or get rid of your television. There is a correlation between television watching and obesity. Each 2-hour increase in daily television watching was associated with a 23% increase in obesity and a 7% increase in diabetes risk. Not surprisingly, television watching is also associated with increased incidence of Alzheimer's disease.[67] Life is short – live it!

---

[67] Science v. 300, No. 5618, p421, 4/18/03; Science v. 309, No. 5736, p 864, 8/5/05

DAY 6: 10-MINUTE WORKOUT
(Descriptions on DAY 2)
Repeat each exercise 30-40 times, and remember to breathe.

Calves-Straight-Toe Raise

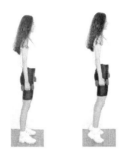

Quadriceps/Glut-Squat

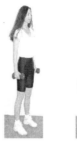
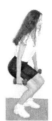

Hamstring-Lunge

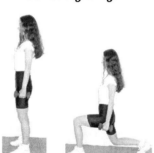

Abdominal-Crunch

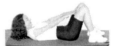
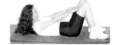

Abdominal-Leg Lowering

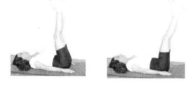

EXTRA EXERCISE:
Abdominal-Alternate Twist

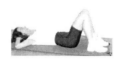
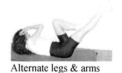

Alternate legs & arms

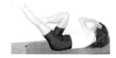

ANSWER YOUR DREAM QUESTION:

6. *Suppose you could spend a fantasy month living someone else's life. They may be alive now or a historical figure. You can choose either a particular person, such as Cleopatra, or a person's role, such as an astronaut or the President of the United States. (A) State the person or role and describe how you imagine the month would play out. (B) What would be the most exciting and wonderful aspect or experience of your fantasy month?*

(A) _____

_____

_____

_____

_____

_____

_____

(B) _____

_____

_____

_____

_____

_____

WORDS FOR THOUGHT

For we are his workmanship, created in Christ Jesus unto good works, which God hath before ordained that we should walk in them. Ephesians 2:10.

Whether therefore ye eat, or drink, or whatsoever ye do, do all to the glory of God. I Corinthians 10:31.

SLEEP 7 TO 8 HOURS

DAY 7

Record your weight_____ lbs.

 Suggested menu – Portions are for one person. Double, triple, etc., for more people. Adjust portions according to height and body type. Weigh yourself to see that you are losing weight at a reasonable rate and adjust accordingly.

Breakfast: Oatmeal and Yogurt and Fruit

- 1 cup cooked oatmeal with 5 walnut or pecan halves and cinnamon
- 1 cup plain organic yogurt mixed with 1 cup blueberries or other fruit
- Vegetable juice or unsweetened fruit juice
- Herbal or green tea or coffee

Lunch: Stuffed Pita Bread

- Pita bread (use regular whole grain bread if you cannot find pita bread) stuffed with:
  > ½ to ¾ cup humus or mashed tofu, tempeh, albacore tuna, or wild salmon mixed with 2 to 3 tablespoons of plain yogurt, ginger, turmeric, and a generous amount of spinach and tomatoes.
- A pear or seasonal fruit
- Water or herbal tea

2:30 PM Snack:

- Orange or peach and carrot sticks. Drink plenty of water.

Evening: (If necessary)

- 1 cup juice, soymilk, or warm milk/soymilk with cinnamon and nutmeg

Tip: *During your old dinnertime, go to a bookstore or library or search the internet for articles, magazines, and books on the subjects that you may truly find fascinating and could lead to a more meaningful and exciting future. Ponder the "Dream Questions" and investigate how to begin the adventure of living them.*

DAY 7: 10-MINUTE WORKOUT

(Descriptions on DAY 1)
Repeat each exercise 30-40 times, and remember to breathe.

Biceps—Curl

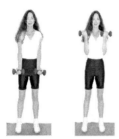

Shoulders--Side Raise

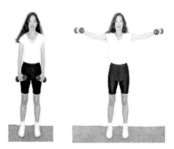

Back--Bent Lift

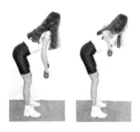

Triceps--Pushback

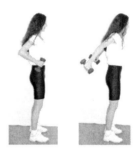

Chest-Push-Ups

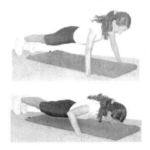

ALTERNATE: Chest-Bench Press

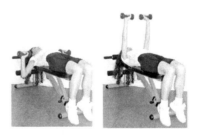

ANSWER YOUR DREAM QUESTION:

7. *Imagine you could go back to an earlier time in your life and tell yourself to change something. (A) What time would that be and what change would you suggest to your younger self? (B) How would your life be different today based on making that change?*

(A) _____

_____

_____

_____

_____

_____

_____

(B) _____

_____

_____

_____

_____

_____

_____

_____

WORDS FOR THOUGHT

And we know that all things work together for good to them that love God, to them who are the called according to His purpose. Romans 8:28.

Lay not up for yourselves treasures upon earth, where moth and rust doth corrupt, and where thieves break through and steal: But lay up for yourselves treasures in heaven, where neither moth nor rust doth corrupt, and where thieves do not break through nor steal. Matthew 6:19-20.

SLEEP 7 TO 8 HOURS

DAY 8

Record your weight_____lbs.

Suggested menu – Portions are for one person. Double, triple, etc., for more people. Adjust portions according to height and body type. Weigh yourself to see that you are losing weight at a reasonable rate and adjust accordingly.

Breakfast: "On the Go" Cottage Cheese Nut Butter Blend and Fruit (Or Cottage Cheese Danish)

- Stir 2 tablespoons tahini or other nut or seed butter into 1 cup organic cottage cheese.

(*Or* substitute Day 3 Breakfast: Cottage Cheese Danish)

- Apple or seasonal fruit
- Herbal or green tea, coffee, and/or low-sugar fruit or vegetable juice

Lunch: Steamed (raw, or stir-fried) Veggies
Makes two servings for Day 8 and Day 9 Lunches - eat half

- Steam about 2 cups of vegetables (broccoli, cauliflower, etc.) and add:
    2 cup cooked rice noodles,
    1 cup tempeh, fish (albacore tuna or wild salmon), or tofu,
    tamari sauce, turmeric, ginger, favorite spices,
    1 tablespoon olive oil, flaxseed oil, *or* nut butter.
    (Option to prepare as stir-fry or have raw as salad.)
- Water or herbal tea

2:30 PM Snack:

- Vegetable or unsweetened fruit juice and drink plenty of water

Evening: (If necessary)

- 1 cup juice, soymilk, or warm milk/soymilk with cinnamon and nutmeg

Tip: It is easier to not begin eating dinner than to push yourself away from the table once you have started. Providing you have satisfied your hunger in a healthy way earlier in the day, it is unlikely your body needs a meal at night.

DAY 8: 10-MINUTE WORKOUT

(Descriptions on DAY 2)
Repeat each exercise 30-40 times, and remember to breathe.

Calves-Straight-Toe Raise

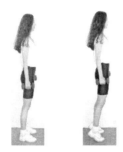

Quadriceps/Glut-Squat

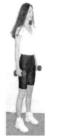
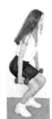

Hamstring-Lunge

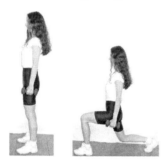

Abdominal-Crunch

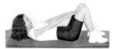
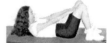

Abdominal-Leg Lowering

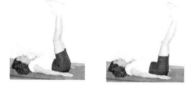

EXTRA EXERCISE:
Abdominal-Alternate Twist

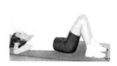

Alternate legs & arms

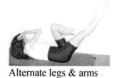

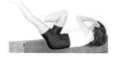

ANSWER YOUR DREAM QUESTION:

8. Carefully read your answers to Dream Questions 1 through 7. (A) What do they say to you in general? (B) What do they say about your dreams and aspirations? (C) List 3 things that surprise you about your answers when you look at them in totality.

(A) _____

_____

_____

_____

_____

_____

(B) _____

_____

_____

_____

_____

_____

(C)1. _____

2. _____

3. _____

_____

WORDS FOR THOUGHT

For where your treasure is, there will your heart be also. Matthew 6:21.

And thine ears shall hear a word behind thee, saying, This is the way, walk ye in it, when ye turn to the right hand, and when ye turn to the left. Isaiah 30:21.

SLEEP 7 TO 8 HOURS

DAY 9

Record your weight_____lbs.

Suggested menu – Portions are for one person. Double, triple, etc., for more people. Adjust portions according to height and body type. Weigh yourself to see that you are losing weight at a reasonable rate and adjust accordingly.

Breakfast: Granola, Yogurt, and Fruit

- ½ to 1 cup granola with rice milk (or other milk)
- 1 cup plain organic yogurt mixed with 1 cup strawberries or other fruit
- Grapefruit or unsweetened juice
- Herbal or green tea or cup of coffee

Lunch: Steamed (or raw, or stir-fried) Veggies
Second half of Day 8's lunch
(Enjoy not having to prepare lunch today!)

- Second day of Day 8's lunch
- Water or herbal tea

2:30 PM Snack:

- Apple, pear, or seasonal fruit and drink plenty of water

Evening: (If necessary)

- 1 cup juice, soymilk, or warm milk/soymilk with cinnamon and nutmeg

Tip: *Eating nutritiously early in the day and not eating after 3:00 PM is the* **secret** *to sustained weight control and therefore better health.*

DAY 9: 10-MINUTE WORKOUT
(Descriptions on DAY 1)
Repeat each exercise 30-40 times, and remember to breathe.

Biceps—Curl

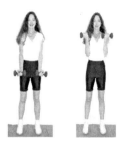

Shoulders--Side Raise

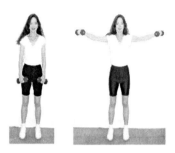

Back--Bent Lift

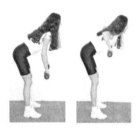

Triceps--Pushback

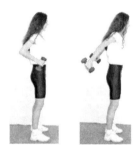

Chest-Push-Ups

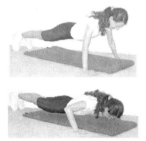

ALTERNATE: Chest-Bench Press

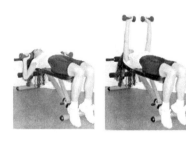

ANSWER YOUR DREAM QUESTION:

9. (A) List 5 dreams or goals you want to pursue further as possible additions to your life. (B) Describe your dream life. (C) Describe the body you need to assist you in living that dream life.

(A)1. _____

2. _____

3. _____

4. _____

5. _____

(B) _____

_____

_____

_____

_____

_____

(C) _____

_____

_____

_____

_____

WORDS FOR THOUGHT

If any of you lack wisdom, let him ask of God, that giveth to all men liberally, and upbraideth not; and it shall be given him. James 1:5.

What? know ye not that your body is the temple of the Holy Ghost which is in you, which ye have of God, and ye are not your own? For ye are bought with a price: therefore glorify God in your body, and in your spirit, which are God's. I Corinthians 6:19-20.

SLEEP 7 TO 8 HOURS

DAY 10

Record your weight_____lbs.

Suggested menu – Portions are for one person. Double, triple, etc., for more people. Adjust portions according to height and body type.

Breakfast: "Late for Work" Yogurt Nut Butter Blend and Fruit

- *Stir 3 tablespoons almond butter (or other nut or seed butter) into 1 cup organic plain yogurt*
- *1 cup blueberries or seasonal fruit*
- *Herbal or green tea, coffee, and/or low-sugar fruit or vegetable juice*

Lunch: Vegetable Bean Salad OR Stuffed Pita Bread

- *Vegetable salad: 1 cup romaine, broccoli, cucumber, radishes, cauliflower, etc. Add ½ to 1 cup black beans or garbanzo beans, 7 walnut or pecan halves, 1 tablespoon flaxseed or olive oil, lemon juice, turmeric, and ginger.*

OR

- *Pita bread (use regular whole grain bread if you cannot find pita bread) stuffed with: ½ to ¾ cup humus or mashed tofu, tempeh, albacore tuna, or wild salmon mixed with 2 to 3 tablespoons of plain yogurt, ginger, turmeric, and a generous amount of spinach and tomatoes.*

- *A pear or seasonal fruit*
- *Water or herbal tea*

2:30 PM Snack:

- *Vegetable juice and drink plenty of water*

Evening: (If necessary)

- *1 cup juice, soymilk, or warm milk/soymilk with cinnamon and nutmeg*

Tip: Focus your evenings on the activities and pursuits that give your life meaning.

DAY 10: 10-MINUTE WORKOUT

(Descriptions on DAY 2)
Repeat each exercise 30-40 times, and remember to breathe.

Calves-Straight-Toe Raise

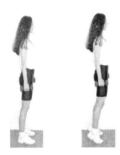

Quadriceps/Glut-Squat

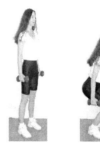

Hamstring-Lunge

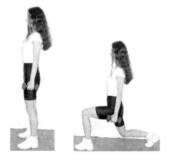

Abdominal-Crunch

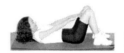

Abdominal-Leg Lowering

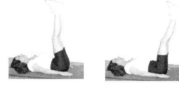

EXTRA EXERCISE:
Abdominal-Alternate Twist

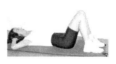
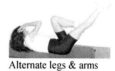

Alternate legs & arms

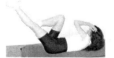

ANSWER YOUR DREAM QUESTION:

10. (A) *Make a plan: Describe how you will investigate pursuing your dreams. (For example, list steps to do to learn more about your prospective interests; browse relevant books and magazines in the library, bookstores, and internet; and borrow or buy relevant books and magazine subscriptions. Then see what holds your attention – what do you really end up reading and learning about?) (B) Describe in detail how will go about changing your body in order to fully live your dream life?*

(A) _____

_____

_____

_____

_____

_____

_____

(B) _____

_____

_____

_____

_____

_____

_____

WORDS FOR THOUGHT

I can do all things through Christ which strengtheneth me. Philippians 4:13.

Brethren, I count not myself to have apprehended: but this one thing I do, forgetting those things which are behind, and reaching forth unto those things which are before, I press toward the mark for the prize of the high calling of God in Christ Jesus. Philippians 3:13-14.

SLEEP 7 TO 8 HOURS

Tomorrow morning - take your final weight and record _____ lbs.

Alternate Breakfast and Lunch

Following are suggestions for an alternate breakfast and lunch that can be substituted for any day(s) of the Dream Diet. You may also use these as suggestions as you continue with 3:00 PM days beyond your first ten days.

Breakfast: Old Fashioned Muesli

- *Old Fashioned Muesli (2 servings): Mix together*
    1 cup uncooked quick 1-minute oats,
    ¼ cup wheat germ,
    ¼ cup chopped nuts
    ¾ cup soy or rice milk,
    ¼ cup orange juice
    Optional ¼ cup raisins
    Cover and let sit overnight or for 8 hours in refrigerator.
    Add rice or soy milk if needed before eating.
- *1 cup blueberries or seasonal fruit*
- *Vegetable juice.*

Lunch: Oven-roasted vegetables

- *Oven-roasted vegetables:*
    Mix vegetables (squash, peppers, etc.) with 2 tablespoons olive oil,
    add ginger, turmeric and other herbs and
    roast as you would for oven roasting vegetables.
    Add 1 tablespoon sesame seeds and
    ½ to ¾ cup tempeh or fish (albacore, wild salmon, etc.)
- *Water or herbal tea*

Chapter 4

Lifestyle Secrets and Inspirations from Alaska to the World

By
Isabelle and Trevor

"Testing. Is this little recorder working? Oh. Hi. It's me, Isabelle here on a beautiful **Alaska** mountaintop with my husband, Trevor. We spend a lot of our time in Alaska and love to hike up as many mountain peaks as possible. We want to live long and healthy lives and have studied nutrition and lifestyle practices that will help us remain young and vibrant as we age. We have noticed there is much nutritional wisdom that has bubbled up from various parts of the world – and there seems to be a pattern. So we did some research and want to share what we discovered. As we stand here on top of South Suicide Peak in the Chugach Mountains overlooking Anchorage, Alaska on this lovely summer day, we want to take you on a virtual trip around the world beginning in our favorite place, Alaska!"

Trevor and Isabelle had just hiked from sea level along Turnagain Arm to over 5,000 feet, and were pleased to find the rocky peak sunny and almost warm. They brought their notes and a recorder.

Trevor spoke into the microphone. "Be careful to shield the microphone from wind gusts. I'll hold our notes flat so we can both see them. I'm not sure doing a recording up here was a great idea, but the views are stunning! I really wish everyone could have a mountaintop experience like this!"

They selected this particular peak in the Chugach Mountains because it gave them a "top-of-the-world" feeling with great 360 degree views. Isabelle was the one who first thought of a nutritional world tour and

Trevor suggested hiking to a place from which they felt they could almost see around the world to add some drama. It had not occurred to him that South Suicide Peak was an odd place to discuss longevity. They felt at home on the peak, surrounded by other high points they had visited on earlier expeditions: O'Malley, Ptarmigan, The Ramp, Avalanche, Bird Ridge Overlook, and McHugh.

"What I like about these health and longevity studies," Isabelle began, "is that they don't just involve controlled experiments in labs. The incredible health and longer life spans of some groups of people have attracted attention. The obvious question was – how do they do it?"

"Right," Trevor added. "And what was discovered is that it wasn't good genes, good climate, or anything unique to a particular place. It was nutrition and lifestyle. In other words, we each have the opportunity to import health and longevity from around the world right into our home." He paused. "So honey, where do we begin?" He tilted the microphone toward Isabelle.

"Great!" Isabelle cleared her throat. "Let's begin our nutrition chronicle right here in Alaska with Alaska Natives, who are obviously very smart and industrious, considering they have survived brutally cold Alaska winters for generations."

"Not only did they survive the winters," Trevor added, glancing at their research notes, "but they have had an enviably low prevalence of health problems, including insulin resistance, metabolic syndrome, and diabetes. Scientists say it's due to their high-omega-3 traditional diet."

"Yes, Trevor," Isabelle said, enjoying their role playing as science teachers. "Scientists have learned by observing Alaska Natives that consuming a lot of omega-3 fatty acids found in fish is protective against metabolic syndrome, insulin sensitivity, and glucose intolerance."[68]

"That's right." Trevor scanned their notes. "The traditional diet of Alaska Natives, rich in omega-3 fatty fish and marine mammals such as seal, walrus, and whale, has also provided these wise individuals with lower *death rates from cardiovascular disease. In fact, an autopsy-based study found that Alaska Natives had lower coronary artery atherosclerosis, which researchers attributed to their high dietary intake of omega-3 fatty acids. They think this lower coronary artery atherosclerosis – did I pronounce that right? – contributes to their lower death rate from heart disease."[69]*

"There has been a lot of research suggesting that omega-3 fats protect against cardiovascular disease." Isabelle stopped momentarily and looked across an ocean of ice-capped peaks.

"What is interesting, Isabelle, is that as Alaska Natives have moved away from their traditional foods to eat a more 'Western' diet, their prevalence of diabetes has rapidly increased. Unfortunately, their incidence of glucose intolerance and insulin resistance is also on the rise."[70]

"Not only are they eating less omega-3's, but modern commercial diets are also laced with sugar."

"You're right, Isabelle. A recent study of a subpopulation of Alaska Natives revealed that they have a diet consisting of both traditional Native foods and store-bought foods. The good news is that their intake of omega-3 fats from fish and sea mammals was still over twenty times greater than the general U.S. population. Unfortunately, they are also consuming an excess of simple sugars, which is likely to be contributing to a rise in obesity and diabetes. They are also deficient in fruits and vegetables. Researchers are recommending they emphasize the positive aspects of Native foods and also increase consumption of fruits and veggies.[71]

"And stop eating commercial sugary foods!" Isabelle declared.

"Amen, Isabelle! That's good advice for everyone! I also might add that in another study on the impact of a more modern Western diet on Alaska Natives, researchers found that Natives who still consume a greater proportion of traditional Native foods, especially omega-3 fats, had better

[68] International Journal of Circumpolar Health v.64, No.4, p.396-408, Sep 2005

[69] Atherosclerosis v.181, No.2, p.353-62, Aug 2005

[70] International Journal of Circumpolar Health v.58, No.2, p.108-19, Apr 1999

[71] *International Journal of Circumpolar Health v.68, No.2, p.109-22, Apr 2009*

fatty acid blood profiles (with more 'good' high-density lipoprotein cholesterol and less 'bad' triglycerides) resulting in better cardiovascular health.[72]

Isabelle looked eastward toward a distant, stunning ice field and then turned a page in their notebook. "Another country that has contributed to our knowledge of the benefits of omega-3 fats is **Greenland.** The low incidence and death rates from cardiovascular disease among Greenland Inuit Natives also spawned much research beginning in the 1970s into whether a high consumption of omega-3 fish fats could prevent heart disease."

"Yes, observations of Greenland Natives and heart disease has generated countless studies exploring the effects of omega-3 fatty acids." Now it was Trevor's turn to be distracted. He pulled his 50-x binoculars out of his daypack to get a close-up view of the distant ice field that had caught Isabelle's attention. "Awesome!"

Isabelle continued, "I read that consuming omega-3 rich fish over long periods of time not only prevents atherosclerosis, but it can reduce rates of sudden cardiac death.[73] Further studies demonstrated a 40% reduction in sudden cardiac deaths in patients after heart attacks if they were treated with at least 1 gram omega-3 fatty acids daily, either by consumption of fish twice weekly or omega-3 fatty acids in capsules. These findings led to recommendations by the American Heart Association and the European Society of Cardiology for daily intake of 1 gram omega-3 fatty acids as a prevention of cardiovascular diseases."[74]

"That's huge, Isabelle! I also read that people who have experienced a heart attack can decrease their death rates if they take 1 gram of omega-3's daily. Furthermore, omega-3's have demonstrated potent anti-inflammatory

---

[72] Journal of the American Dietetic Association v.108, No.2, p.266-73, Feb 2008

[73] Current Vascular Pharmacology v.6, No.1, p.1, Jan 2008

[74] Herz. v.31, Suppl 3, p.24-30, Dec 2006

effects.[75] Check out the glaciers hanging off that ice field out there!" Trevor said, pointing and handing Isabelle the binoculars.

Isabelle took the binoculars and steadied herself against a rock. She took a long look at the massive ice field and glaciers. "I am always amazed how blue glaciers are – it's just so beautiful!"

Isabelle lowered the binoculars and gave Trevor a serious look. "From Greenland Natives, to **Japanese** fishing villages, and beyond – there is so much evidence that what we eat really matters. Just eating fish oil can protect against coronary heart disease and atherosclerosis. It's amazing! In fact, the beneficial effects of fish oil are mostly attributed to their omega-3 fatty acids, eicosapentaenoic acid (EPA) and docosahexaenoic acid (DHA)."[76] She enunciated these impressive names very carefully.

Trevor was taken by how serious Isabelle was about nutrition and exercise. "I am fortunate to be married to someone so knowledgeable who wants to take such good care of me!"

Isabelle laughed at her earnest tone. "OK. I know I'm a bit over the top. I just want people to understand how important this information is. For example, having a diet low in omega-3's and high in animal proteins, saturated fats, and commercial omega-6 vegetable oils is associated with a higher incidence of cardiovascular disease, certain cancers, and autoimmune disorders such as rheumatoid arthritis, Systemic Lupus Erythematosus, and renal disease. Conversely, increasing intake of omega-3's decreases the severity of autoimmune disorders, lessens the chance of developing cardiovascular disease, and protects against bone loss during post-menopause.[77]

Trevor shifted his position on their high perch and trained the binoculars on a distant turquoise glacial lake. Rather than taking his eyes off the lake and its surreal color, he spoke from memory. "You mentioned

[75] QJM v.96, No.7, p.465-80 Jul 2003; Panminerva Medica v.45, No.2, p.99-07, Jun 2003; Mayo Clinic Proceedings v.75, No.6, p.607-14, Jun 2000

[76] Journal of Nutritional Biochemistry v.19, No.7, p.417-37, Jul 2008

[77] Frontiers in Bioscience v.13, p.4015, 5/1/2008

the DHA *fatty acid in fish oil, Isabelle. Did you know that research in* **China** *showed that higher fish consumption correlated with higher levels of DHA in red blood cells, lower levels of blood triglyceride concentrations, and lower incidence of cardiovascular disease?"*[78]

Isabelle *was also staring down at the turquoise lake. "Wow. From Alaska and Greenland Natives to Japan and China – they teach us the benefits of consuming omega-3's."*

"Speaking of **Japan** *and* **China***, Isabelle, I'm sure you know that the incidences of breast and prostate cancers are much higher in the United States and European countries than in Japan and China."*

"That's right, Trevor, and one of the major differences in diet is that the Japanese and Chinese consume a traditional diet high in soy." Isabelle *became animated. "In fact, the soy compounds called isoflavones or phytoestrogens are believed to play a role in reducing the incidence of breast and prostate cancers. In particular, the soy phytoestrogen, genistein, has been shown in animal studies to inhibit cancer formation. Researchers think genistein targets the estrogen sites in the processes of cancer formation, and interferes with cancer development. Various studies have provided evidence that the soy-component genistein is a promising cancer fighter."*[79]

Now Trevor *referred back to their notes. "You're right. The phytoestrogens, genistein and daidzein, found in soy, can bind to estrogen receptors and therefore interfere with the action of estrogen, which is a well-established risk factor for breast, ovarian, and endometrial cancers. Although not all results are consistent, there is good evidence for the protective influence of soy foods against all three of these cancers. There have also been many reports of soy's preventive effects on the prostate."*[80] Trevor *stood up and walked over to view the slice of Anchorage they could see beyond McHugh and Ptarmigan peaks.*

---

[78] Comparative Biochemistry and Physiology: A Molecular Integrative Physiology v.136, No.1, p.127-40, Sep 2003

[79] Cancer Investigation v.21, No.5, p.744-57, 2003

[80] Asian Pacific Journal of Cancer Prevention v.9, No.4, p.543-8, Oct-Dec 2008

Isabelle followed Trevor with notes and recorder in hand. "Yes, Trevor. And what's interesting is that when Asian women migrate to the United States, their breast cancer risk increases and approaches that for U.S. women."

"I guess that's due to adopting a Western diet," Trevor suggested.

"Exactly. And furthermore, a study of women of Asian descent living in the U.S. revealed that soy intake during childhood, adolescence, and adult life was associated with decreased breast cancer risk.[81]

Trevor moved dangerously close to the vertical north face and aimed his binoculars down at Rabbit Lake, a few thousand feet below them. "Honey, Japan has the longest life expectancy in the world. But, as their diet becomes more Westernized, the number of people with metabolic syndrome, diabetes, cardiovascular disease, and cerebrovascular diseases keeps increasing."[82]

"It's ridiculous that human beings seem to have such a propensity to self destruct by eating sugar, red meat, and unhealthy fats! Speaking of self-destructive behavior, please get away from that cliff! I don't think you would glide very well!"

Trevor just smiled and returned to the rock they had been sitting on and reclined on one elbow. "You won't lose me that easily, Isabelle." He looked at the notes and continued. "Now, people in **Okinawa** have had the highest longevity rates in Japan and possess healthy cardiovascular systems even at advanced ages. This has been linked to their plant-based diet high in vegetables and soy, low in salt, and with monounsaturates as the principal fat. They also get regular physical activity and have minimal tobacco use. Not surprisingly, they have a low incidence of breast, ovary, prostate, and colon cancers and low rates of hip fractures.[83] In fact, due to their moderate intake of calories, researchers suggest that older Okinawans provide an interesting population study of people who may have undergone a mild form

---

[81] Cancer Epidemiology, Biomarkers & Prevention v.18, No.4, p.1050-9, Apr 2009

[82] Yakugaku Zasshi v.127, No.3, p.399-406, Mar 2007

[83] Asia Pacific Journal of Clinical Nutrition v.10, No.2, p.165-71, 2001

of prolonged caloric restriction for about half their adult lives, which may have contributed to their extended lifespans and lowered risk for age-associated chronic diseases."[84]

Isabelle looked into Trevor's eyes. "Unfortunately, recent life expectancy data for Okinawan men was no higher than the national Japanese average. Researchers believe this decline in longevity among Okinawans is due to increased heart disease and cerebrovascular disease that occurred with a movement away from their traditional diet high in pulses – uh, beans, peas, etcetera – and vegetables.[85]

Isabelle leaned over and kissed Trevor on the cheek. She then sat up straight and took in her favorite view of the distant ice fields and glaciers atop the Kenai Peninsula. "You know, Trevor, we really need to mention the **Mediterranean** diet. It has been inspired by the traditional diets of countries of the Mediterranean basin. Of course, diets vary among these countries." She consulted the notes. "Nevertheless, there are certain characteristics that make up what is referred to as the Mediterranean diet such as: high in fruits, vegetables, nuts, olive oil, beans, legumes, and cereals; moderate to high in fish; moderate in alcohol; low to moderate in dairy products; and low in red meat, processed meat, meat products, eggs, and refined carbohydrates.[86]

Trevor felt a chilled wind gust, put his arm around Isabelle's shoulders, and looked across the sea of ice-capped peaks. "People who adhere to the principles of the traditional Mediterranean diet tend to have a longer lifespan and a lower incidence of heart disease. And we should point out that these people are also more physically active."[87]

"We're certainly physically active," Isabelle mused, looking down at her well-worn hiking boots. "And I might add there sure are benefits to following a traditional Mediterranean diet – reduced risk of metabolic

---

[84] Biogerontology v.7, No.3, p173-7, Jun 2006

[85] Asia Pacific Journal of Public Health v.15, Suppl:S3-9, 2003

[86] Harefuah v.147, No.5 p.422-7, 477, May 2008; Maturitas Aug 31 2009; Maturitas Aug 31 2009; BMJ v.338, No.b2337. Jun 23 2009

[87] Harefuah v.147, No.5 p.422-7, 477, May 2008; Maturitas Aug 31 2009; BMJ v.338, No.b2337. Jun 23 2009

syndrome, high blood pressure, cardiovascular disease, death after a heart attack, obesity, cancer, diseases related to chronic inflammation, rheumatoid arthritis, and neurodegenerative age-related diseases such as dementia, Alzheimer's disease, Parkinson's disease.[88]

Trevor pointed to a pair of ravens perched on a protruding rock below them. "I read that the longevity of Mediterranean people has been largely credited to olive oil and vegetables.[89]

"That's right. And olive oil and other healthy fats are thought to be protective against upper digestive tract cancers as well as breast, ovarian, and colorectal cancer. Whole grain foods also may reduce the risk of upper digestive tract and various other cancers. In contrast, refined grain intake and high glycemic index foods may increase the risk for several cancers. As we've discussed, fish and omega-3 fatty acids are extremely beneficial, while frequent red meat intake has been directly related to some common cancers.[90] *There are few things people can do to themselves worse than eating processed meats and red meat!" Isabelle said with passion.*

"Right on, Isabelle! And interestingly the beneficial aspects of the Mediterranean diet are many of the same dietary principles that have increased lifespan and reduced disease in other parts of the world." Trevor snuggled closer to Isabelle as the sun hid behind a scudding cloud. They held the recorder together.

"You're right, Trevor. Like low consumption of meat and meat products and high consumption of vegetables, fruits, nuts, legumes, beans, and healthy monounsaturated and omega-3 fats from olive oil, nuts, and fish."[91]

"Yeah, and we can add to the 'healthy list' moderate or modest wine consumption."[92]

---

[88] Maturitas Aug 31 2009; Public Health Nutrition v.12, No.9A, p.1607-17, Sep 2009; Public Health Nutrition v.12, No.9A, p.1595-600, Sep 2009

[89] Maturitas Aug 31 2009

[90] Public Health Nutrition v.12, No. 9A, p.1595-600, Sept 2009

[91] BMJ v.338, No.b2337. Jun 23 2009; Public Health Nutrition v.12, No. 9A, p.1595-600, Sept 2009

[92] BMJ v.338, No.b2337. Jun 23 2009

"*Moving a bit to the north,*" *Isabelle sighed,* "*a study estimated that more than 1 in 3 men and 1 in 4 women age 75 and over are living with coronary heart disease in the* **UK**. *What do you think the researchers' recommendations are? I know what you're thinking! A diet high in fruits, vegetables, whole-grains, oily fish (omega-3's), and low in saturated fat. They say that such diets, together with regular physical activity, avoidance of smoking, sensible drinking habits, and maintenance of a healthy body weight may prevent the majority of cardiovascular disease in Western populations.*"[93]

"*More confirmation of the same,*" *Trevor smiled at Isabelle.* "*Stay slim, get vigorous exercise, and eat the right foods! Not to mention being in love.*"

"*I like that!*" *Isabelle gave Trevor another kiss on the cheek.* "*And speaking of the 'right' foods,*" *Isabelle pointed toward the southeast.* "*There are certain foods, sometimes called 'super foods' or 'nutraceuticals', which are packed with antioxidants and healthy compounds. For example, some researchers at the University of São Paulo in* **Brazil** *reported that healthy foods and nutraceuticals hold great promise for improving health and fighting age-related diseases, cancer, cardiovascular disease, and neurodegenerative diseases. They said bioactive compounds from different foods, herbs, and nutraceuticals (such as ginseng, nuts, grains, tomato, soy phytoestrogens, curcumin, melatonin, polyphenols, antioxidant vitamins, carnitine, carnosine, and ubiquinone) can help or even prevent diseases.*"[94]

"*That's a mouthful,*" *Trevor laughed.*

"*You better believe it!*" *Isabelle pulled a small plastic bag from her jacket pocket containing six wild blueberries.* "*Here, honey, have your neutraceuticals. I picked these earlier before we began the steep part of our climb.*"

"*Hey, wild blueberries – my favorite!*" *Trevor began savoring them one by one.*

---

[93] British Journal of Community Nursing v.14, No.5, p.210, May 2009

[94] Biogerontology v.5, No.5, p.275-89, 2004

*Isabelle felt the wind pick up and thought she felt a small drop of rain on her cheek. "Do you know what **India's** gold is, Trevor?"*

"I know India is a big consumer of gold jewelry, but I don't think that's what you're referring to," Trevor said with a half smile.

"You're right. I'm talking about curcumin, which gives the golden color to turmeric. It has been shown to exhibit antioxidant, anti-inflammatory, anticancer, antiviral, antibacterial, antifungal, and anti-atherosclerotic activities and may be helpful in fighting various cancers, diabetes, allergies, arthritis, Alzheimer's disease, and other chronic illnesses. It has also been found to increase detoxifying enzymes, prevent DNA damage, improve DNA repair, decrease mutations and tumor formation, and even delay induced cataracts."[95]

"I knew traditional Indian spices had health benefits, such as fenugreek seeds can reduce blood sugar and lipids and may be helpful in diabetes. Similarly garlic, onions, and ginger may help fight cancer." He noticed a few drops of water on their notes.

"That's right, Trevor. In fact, curcumin from turmeric has been reported to be helpful against leukemia and lymphoma, gastrointestinal cancers, genitourinary cancers, breast cancer, ovarian cancer, head and neck squamous cell carcinoma, lung cancer, melanoma, neurological cancers, and sarcoma.[96] And of course there are traditional Indian medical uses of turmeric too, such as in wound healing, rheumatic disorders, gastrointestinal symptoms, deworming, and rhinitis.[97]

"Wow. Pretty impressive, Isabelle. I'm totally in favor of deworming!"

Isabelle smiled. "And – you're impressed with all that turmeric can do?"

"I am, but I'm mostly impressed with you, Isabelle. By the way, didn't I read about turmeric fighting Alzheimer's disease?"

---

[95] Advanced Experimental Med Biol v.595, p.1-75, 2007; Asia Pacific Journal of Clinical Nutrition v.17, Suppl 1, p.265-8, 2008
[96] Cancer Letters v.267, No.1, p.133-64, 8/18/2008
[97] Asia Pacific Journal of Clinical Nutrition v.17, Suppl 1, p.265-8, 2008

"Yes Trevor. There is a lot of ongoing research on the use of turmeric's curcumin to fight Alzheimer's disease."[98]

Trevor wondered if they should begin gathering their belongings and start down the mountain. He glanced at the notes and spoke a little faster. "But it's not just turmeric's curcumin and the omega-3's we mentioned earlier that benefit our brains and cognitive function. Exercise has been shown to be just as important! Studies show exercise enhances learning and memory.[99] In fact, evidence is accumulating that exercise has profound benefits for brain function. An active lifestyle can prevent or delay loss of cognitive function as we age. Recent research indicates that the effects of exercise on the brain can be enhanced by regular consumption of nutritional compounds such as omega fatty acids or plant polyphenols (like curcumin). There appears to be a synergistic effect between diet and exercise such that optimal maintenance of brain health might depend on both exercise and nutrition.[100] I guess I am just a little passionate about exercise." Trevor noticed he had been speaking more loudly.

Consulting their notes he continued, "But there's more, Isabelle. In a study of people ages 65 to 84 there was a direct correlation between healthy lifestyle and better memory performance. People with the 'healthiest lifestyle' had a low BMI of under 22 and a diet high in fruits, vegetables, whole-grains, and healthy fats. These people also engaged in physical exercise, burning more than 13,000 kcal[101] per week and had a history of never smoking and an alcohol consumption of 4 to 10 drinks per week."[102] Trevor stood up and looked around the rocky peak at the vast beauty surrounding their 5,000 foot mountain and shouted into the wind. "Yes, I am a nut about staying strong and healthy!"

---

[98] Cellular and Molecular Life Sciences v.65, No.11, p.1631-52, Jun 2008; Archives of Physiology and Biochemistry v.114, No.2, p.127-49, Apr 2008; Neuromolecular Medicine v.10, No.4, p.259-74, 2008

[99] Nutrition and Health v.18, No.3, p.277-84, 2006

[100] Trends in Neurosciences v.32, No.5, p.283, May 2009; Neurobiology of Aging v.26, Suppl.1, p.133-6, Dec 2005

[101] Kilocalorie: A unit of heat equal to 1000 calories–the heat required to raise the temperature of 1 kg of H_2O 1°C. McGraw-Hill Concise Dictionary of Modern Medicine

[102] Neuroepidemiology v.31, No.1, p.39-47, 2008

Isabelle giggled. She stood and hugged her husband. "Speaking of nuts, honey, studies have consistently demonstrated the benefits of eating various nuts and peanuts on coronary heart disease.[103] In fact, a high intake of nuts is associated with a 35% reduced risk of coronary heart disease. There is evidence that nut consumption also reduces the risk of diabetes, gallstone diseases,[104] and cancer.[105] Researchers have also suggested that moderate, long-term consumption of nuts is linked with lower body weight and lower risk of obesity and weight gain.[106] In addition to their fatty acids, vitamins, and minerals, nuts and peanuts contain other beneficial bioactive compounds and numerous phytochemicals that promote health and reduce the risk of chronic disease.[107] In fact, researchers believe that if nuts and peanuts were routinely incorporated into a healthy diet, the risk of coronary heart disease would markedly decrease,[108] and that nuts and seeds deserve a separate food group listing in the Dietary Guidelines and should be promoted for good health."[109]

"And what goes with nuts?" Trevor asked.

"Uh, I don't know. Oh. What about fruit?"

"You got it!" He read quickly, "An overwhelming body of research has established that eating berry fruits has a positive and profound impact on human health, performance, and disease. Berries, which are cultivated right here in **North America**, *include blackberry, black raspberry, blueberry, cranberry, red raspberry, and strawberry. Other berry fruits, which are consumed in the* **traditional diets of North American tribal communities**, *include chokecherry, highbush cranberry, serviceberry, and silver buffaloberry. In addition, berry fruits such as arctic bramble, bilberries, black currants, boysenberries, cloudberries, crowberries, elderberries,*

---

[103] Journal of Nutrition v.138, No.9, p.1746-1751, Sep 2008; American Journal of Clinical Nutrition v.89, No.5, p.1643-1648, May 2009

[104] Journal of Nutrition v.138, No.9, p.1763-1765, Sep 2008; American Journal of Clinical Nutrition v.89, No.5, p.1643-1648, May 2009

[105] Asia Pacific Journal of Clinical Nutrition v.17, Suppl 1, p.329-32, 2008

[106] American Journal of Clinical Nutrition v.89, No.5, p.1643-1648, May 2009; Journal of Nutrition v.138, No.9, p.1763-1765, Sep 2008

[107] Journal of Nutrition v.138, No.9, p.1746-1751, Sep 2008; Asia Pacific Journal of Clinical Nutrition v.17, Suppl 1, p.329-32, 2008; Journal of Human Nutrition and Dietetics v.22, No.1, p.64-71, Feb 2009

[108] Journal of Nutrition v.138, No.9, p.1746-1751, Sep 2008

gooseberries, lingonberries, loganberries, marionberries, Rowan berries, and sea buckthorn, are also popularly consumed in other parts of the **world**. *Recently, there has also been a surge in the consumption of exotic berry-type fruits such as the pomegranate, goji berries, mangosteen, and the* **Chilean** *maqui berry."*[110]

"Really?"

"Yes, Isabelle. And growing evidence suggests that flavonoid-rich North American cranberries and blueberries may limit the development and severity of certain cancers and vascular diseases including atherosclerosis, ischemic stroke, and neurodegenerative diseases of aging. In fact, evidence suggests a potential role for dietary cranberry and blueberry in the prevention of cancer and vascular diseases."[111]

"Really? Well, Trevor. Did you know that recent research suggests that dried plums, or prunes, are the most effective fruit in preventing and reversing bone loss? In fact, both animal studies and a 3-month clinical trial have shown that dried plums have positive effects on bone preservation and growth."[112]

"Really? Prunes and bone loss?"

"That's right."

"OK, Isabelle. Here's some dessert to top off our top-of-the mountain, round-the-world nutrition diatribe. Researchers in **Switzerland** *studying coronary heart disease and stroke reported that cocoa demonstrates beneficial effects on blood pressure, insulin resistance, and vascular and platelet function."*[113]

"Really?" Isabelle said with a smile. "I guess we have determined that different cultures have discovered the same wisdom – staying slim, exercise, and nutrition can have a huge impact on your life and health."

---

[109]   Journal of Nutrition v.138, No.9, p.1763S-1765S, Sep 2008

[110]   Journal of Agricultural and Food Chemistry 13;v.56, No.3, p.627-9, Feb 2008

[111]   Molecular Nutrition Food Research v.51, No.6, p.652-64, Jun 2007

[112]   Ageing Res Rev. v.8, No.2, p.122-7, Apr 2009

[113]   Circulation v.119, No.10, p.1433-41, 3/17/2009

"I think you nailed it, Isabelle! But there's one more bit of wisdom I'd like to impart. The sky over there is very dark and we're over three hours from the car – if we move fast. It wouldn't take much rain to turn the lower part of the trail into a slippery mess. Let's see how fast we can get down from here!" Trevor was zipping up his pack.

"Here, honey, don't forget the recorder and notebook. We need to drop them off at Debra's place tonight complete with footnotes. She really wants to finish the book."

With that they began picking their way down the rocky ridge and were soon gliding down the tundra. A family of Dall Sheep observed the visiting bipeds retreat back toward the forest, and then returned to their healthy, natural, green repast.

Chapter 5

What's Next?

It's me, Isabelle, again! Trevor and I made it safely off South Suicide Mountain and congratulations to you for finishing *The Dream Diet!* You did it! You pushed the restart button on your life! You have taken a huge step to freedom from having food run your life. I think by now you realize *The 3:00 PM Secret* lifestyle works and is really very easy. Your future is a blank slate and you can write anything you like on it. It is unwritten and wide open. Go forward and pursue your dream life and dream body!

After following the *Dream Diet* for one or more ten-day periods, you will love the results and will *want* to continue. If you switch back and forth between *The 3:00 PM Secret* lifestyle and your old lifestyle, I believe you will prefer the way you feel on *The Dream Diet* and will slowly adopt it permanently. Once you integrate not eating at night into your life, you will never consider going back to the nightly feeding frenzy, carrying unwanted fat on your body, jeopardizing your health, and feeling lousy. After doing this lifestyle for a period of time, something clicks and your unhealthy desires seem to vanish. You are free from worrying about weight forever!

It is inevitable that you will have special social engagements that will require a dinner party or dining out in a restaurant. You can certainly enjoy these occasions and continue to follow *The 3:00 PM Secret* lifestyle most of the time. When you do eat late at night, you will undoubtedly feel uncomfortable, especially if you eat rich foods. On these occasions, you will find yourself further convinced that eating at night is a mistake. The more you live *The 3:00 PM Secret* lifestyle the more you will want to continue with it since, with very little effort, it will give you a body that is slim, strong, and beautiful.

You may have noticed that people who are able to control their weight over the long term are not necessarily more disciplined or smarter, but instead have simply focused their priorities on life rather than food and have developed good habits. The fact that habits are difficult to break can be a blessing. Once you form good habits and they become ingrained, you will tend to follow and keep them. It is not unusual for us to make major changes in our lifestyle and habits throughout our lives. Eventually we adapt to each new habit, and it becomes programmed into our lives. Once you integrate new, healthy, liberating habits into your life and embark on your long-dreamed-of adventures, you will be an inspiration to family and friends.

Eating a healthy breakfast and lunch and not eating in the late afternoon and evening is the *secret* to sustained weight loss. Adding daily vigorous exercise and 7 to 8 hours of sleep at night will give you the slim, strong body worthy of your dreams and greatly increase your chances of good health, vitality, and an optimistic outlook.

What should you do going forward? Continue to follow the basic tenets of *The 3 PM Secret 10-Day Dream Diet*, create the body worthy of your dreams, find your purpose, and live your dream life. Revisit the *Dream Questions* often and see if your answers change and evolve.

What to Do Going Forward

(1) *Refrain from eating a meal 7 to 9 hours before bedtime.*

(2) *Eat nutritiously. Use the menus for ideas or create your own simple, nutritious meals using the Ten Nutrition Tips in Section 2.4 and What Foods to Focus On and Ideas for Meals later in this chapter. Transfer your focus from food to your dreams!*

(3) *Exercise vigorously for at least ten minutes each day. As you become slimmer and stronger, increase your physical activity. Hike, bike, run, swim, play, etc. I am convinced that vigorous exercise is key to physical and mental health!*

(4) *Sleep 7 to 8 hours each night.*

(5) *Fill in the "Chart Your Future" form on the last page of the book. Review the Dream Questions in Chapter 3 and see if your answers change. Continue to pursue and live your dreams.*

* * * * * * * * * * * * * * * * * * *

MALE MUSING ON TRANSITION

After carefully following *The 3 PM Secret* lifestyle for 10 or more days, stop for a moment and consider what you have discovered. Have you begun to lose weight? Do you feel stronger? Are you more rested? Does it feel good to go to bed without feeling full? Has your stomach stopped demanding to be fed in the evening when you don't need more food? Have you started to believe that maybe you **can** get control over your body?   Stop for a moment and consider these questions, but don't stop for too long!

Why not stop for a while? Because you are swimming against the tide of a lifetime of habits and traditions that will not release their grip in just 10 days – they are too much a part of you. These may habits include regular large evening meals, unhealthy food choices, no regular exercise, too little sleep, and not believing in your dreams.

Regardless of the good progress you have made in the last 10 days, if you stop moving forward, these old habits will relentlessly push you back to where you started. Then they will mock your failure. You may also have comforting friends trying to sabotage your progress with what appear to be acts of kindness.

Changing to a healthy lifestyle is like trying to go up a down escalator. Before you reach the top, if you stop you'll quickly lose all the ground you've gained.

So, you have an important decision to make: Do you continue with your new healthy practices or allow the old habits to regain control of your body? You have learned that you can follow the 3 PM lifestyle - you just did it for 10 days with beneficial effects. The question is: will you choose to continue or will you again give up on seeking a trim, strong, and healthy body? It's your life - how do you want to live it?

We believe that after only 10 days you have discovered, over the protests and whining of the old habits, that you really like the way you're starting to look and feel. If you **dare**, test this by spending the next 10 days having large late dinners, eating primarily unhealthy processed foods, avoiding exercise, and making sure you don't sleep more than 6 hours. After this 10-day period, stop and ask the same questions from the first paragraph. We have no doubt that you will not be happy about feeling stuffed, tired, and alarmed at the huge weight gain! You may not need to actually revert to bad habits if you have a good imagination - you already know what will happen.

Do you need to keep repeating this 10-day program forever? You could, but if you're like me, a little variety would be nice! I suggest you try successive 7 or 10 day versions of the "Dream Diet" (with a day off in between or when needed for special occasions). Modify the details by adding some alternative healthy foods and recipes and also by adding enjoyable physical activities and exercises. Ask family and friends to continue to encourage (and not sabotage) you.

Little by little, within the book's basic guidelines, you will find you have discovered a liberating and healthy lifestyle that will serve you for a lifetime. So long as you eat moderate amounts of nutritious foods, don't eat late in your day, exercise regularly, and sleep enough, you will like the results. Debra's book, "The 3 PM Secret: Live Slim and Strong Live Your Dreams", provides additional information and tools to help you write the recipe for your own happiness and success. Our hope for you is that you will reach the top of the down escalator of destructive habits and then take off after your dreams in a great new slim and fit body. We hope you never stop and never go back to the old habits, and that you take the time to bring along your family and friends! Your future has not yet been written - make it wonderful!

* * * * * * * * * * * * * * * * * * * *

What Foods to Focus On

Following is a list of nourishing foods from the vegetables, fruits, fats, protein, and carbohydrates groups that can be used to make healthy meal choices as you continue to develop your new eating habits. It is not a complete listing of all healthy and nutritious foods, but rather good examples of foods you should consider. It is important to eat whole foods in their natural form rather than processed, packaged, or prepared foods, which are not healthy and are full of empty calories, sugars, artificial sweeteners, unhealthy fats, filler additives, over-processed grains, chemicals, and other potentially dangerous additives.

VEGETABLES:

It is essential to make eating vegetables a daily priority. There are almost endless varieties of vegetables to choose from – some with funny names and shapes. Select from a wide array of vegetables including spinach, broccoli, cabbage, cauliflower, chard, kale, mustard greens, turnips, rutabaga, carrots, beets, radishes, purple cabbage, parsley, asparagus, Brussels sprouts, red and green peppers, various sprouts including bean sprouts and alfalfa sprouts, sea vegetables, red lettuce, cucumbers, celery, asparagus, green beans, eggplant, scallions, onions, garlic, leeks, squash, pumpkin, snow peas, water chestnuts, and artichokes. If you do not have time to wash and prepare fresh vegetables, use pre-washed or frozen vegetables rather than canned. Also, *eat organically grown vegetables whenever possible to avoid ingesting pesticides and other toxic chemicals.*

Vegetables can also be consumed in the form of soups, stews, and fresh vegetable juices. (Juicing books have numerous suggestions for healthy vegetable juices.) It is best if you can make your own soups since most commercially-prepared soups contain unhealthy additives. A second-best alternative is to shop in a health food store or the health food section of a grocery store for healthfully-prepared soups.

FRUIT:

Eat a variety of fruits daily such as grapefruit, oranges, tangerines, lemons, papaya, pineapple, mangos, blueberries, strawberries, raspberries, tomatoes, figs, apricots, peaches, plums, cherries, pears, cantaloupe, grapes, apples, avocados, and bananas. When available, **select organically grown fruit.** You can also drink fresh low-sugar fruit juices such as grapefruit juice. Fruits can be consumed in nutritious shakes and smoothies that are made from various fresh or frozen fruits including blueberries, strawberries, raspberries, peaches, and bananas, as well as nut, soy or rice milk, wheat germ, organic yogurt, and fermented soy, vegetable, or nut powders.

FATS:

Healthy fats contain the essential and beneficial fatty acids and should be part of your daily diet. Foods rich in the important **omega-3 fatty acids** include flaxseed oil, fish oil, cold-water and fatty fish (including salmon, tuna, cod, halibut, and anchovy), as well as fish oil or omega-3 supplements. Other sources of omega-3 fatty acids include pumpkin seeds, walnuts, dark green leafy vegetables, sea vegetables, soybeans, wheat germ, and sprouts. If you do not eat fish several times a week, consider taking omega-3 fatty acid supplements or take one or two tablespoons of flaxseed oil daily. (Note: Store flaxseed oil in the refrigerator.)

Unprocessed olive oil should be used as the primary source of fat in your food preparation. Other beneficial fats are found in foods such as avocados, olives, nuts, seeds, and nut and seed butters. Good quality omega-6 fatty acids are found in raw nuts and seeds, legumes, leafy green vegetables, evening primrose oil, borage oil, black currant seed oil, gooseberry oil, and grapeseed oil. *Avoid processed, hydrogenated grocery store vegetable oils* such as corn, safflower, sunflower, soybean, cottonseed, and sesame oil because they typically contain transfats.

Nuts, seeds, and nut and seed butters contain both healthful fats and protein. There are a variety of nuts and seeds that can be eaten whole or as butters including almonds, pistachios, pecans, walnuts, cashews, hazelnuts, macadamia nuts, pumpkin seeds, sunflower seeds, almond butter, and tahini. Many nutritionists recommend emphasizing raw nuts and seeds.

PROTEIN:

It is important to eat healthy protein. Protein can be obtained from various foods including fish (salmon, cod, haddock, halibut, mackerel, sardines, tuna, trout), nuts, seeds, nut and seed butters, beans, legumes, soybeans and soy foods (such as tempeh, miso or tofu), protein powder drinks using fermented soy, nuts, whey, organic yogurt, and limited amounts of animal protein such as organic cottage cheese and eggs. If you eat dairy or poultry, ***use only organic*** to avoid hormones, antibiotics, and milk from animals fed chemicals or diseased or same-species meat.

Protein-containing foods that also provide complex carbohydrates include lentils, chickpeas, beans, legumes, peas, black beans, navy beans, lima beans, pinto beans, green beans, and wheat germ. Other foods that contain both proteins and complex carbohydrates include sprouts from grains, beans, lentils, seeds, and vegetables.

CARBOHYDRATES:

Complex carbohydrate foods that can be part of a healthy diet include beans, peas and legumes, brown rice, wild rice, basmati rice, unprocessed whole grains (including buckwheat, millet, amaranth, quinoa, barley, rye, spelt, bulgur, whole-grain pumpernickel, wheat grain, and barley grain), corn, yams, oats, sprouted breads, and if you are not sensitive to wheat, wheat kernels, cracked wheat, and cracked wheat bread. Avoid or strictly limit processed carbohydrates. Processed carbohydrates include muffins, pastries, sugary commercial breakfast cereals, pasta, white breads, rolls, bagels, most crackers, cookies, cakes, and most prepared snacks, mixes, and convenience foods.

SUPPLEMENTS:

Talk to your doctor about what supplements you should be taking. If you are primarily a vegetarian, check with your doctor about vitamin B12 and zinc supplements. Also check with your doctor about vitamin D. It is found naturally in salmon and fatty fish, and is made when ultraviolet B from the Sun penetrates your skin. Certain foods, including milk and cereal, are also often fortified with some vitamin D. Vitamin D helps regulate calcium for bones, nerves, and heart.[114] Inadequate vitamin D can cause rickets (soft bones, enlarged hearts) in babies and children, and bone fractures in the elderly, and may be involved in cancer and autoimmune diseases. Vitamin D may have antimicrobial properties, help fight infections and flu,[115] and be protective against multiple sclerosis.[116]

WATER:

Drink at least 8 glasses of water a day. You can also drink herbal and green teas and mineral water. Avoid soft drinks, sugary drinks, and artificial sweeteners.

Ideas for Meals

Does it seem easier to buy and eat packaged, prepared foods? Unfortunately, packaged, prepared foods are nearly always filled with unhealthy ingredients and/or chemical additives. It can be nearly as simple and fast to toss together healthy meals. For example, consider hearty vegetable salads that can be made with avocados, nuts, beans, and other healthy ingredients; fruit salads with yogurt and granola; stir-fries with salmon or tofu; and other easy-to-prepare dishes that you create yourself by mixing a few healthy foods.

The less food you eat, the more important it is that the food be highly nutritious and rich in essential amino acids found in protein, essential fatty acids found in high-quality fats and oils, and vitamins and minerals found in vegetables and other whole foods. The idea is to give yourself all the nutrients you need without adding empty calories from foods that are processed, fried, or laden with sugars, unhealthy fats, and toxic additives.

The 3:00 PM Secret lifestyle is not a food-focused existence, but rather a life focused on living your dreams. Following are ideas for what you can include in breakfasts, lunches, and snacks, but be creative according to your own tastes.

---

[114] Science v. 302, No. 5652, p.1886, 12/12/03

[115] FASEB Journal July 2005/Science News v. 170, No.20, 11/11/06

[116] JAMA v.296:2832-2838, 2006, http://jama.ama-assn.org/cgi/content/abstract/296/23/2832;;
J. of the American Dietetic Assoc 2006 03, v.106, Issue 3 http://www.adajournal.org/article/PIIS0002822305020845/pdf

Suggestions to include in Breakfasts. Many of these are described in the Chapter 3 menus:

- Granola or whole grain cereal with rice, soy, or nut milk.
- Plain organic yogurt mixed with strawberries, blueberries, or other fruit.
- Oatmeal with walnut or pecan halves and cinnamon.
- Cottage Cheese Danish: 2 pieces of toast spread with organic cottage cheese mixed with cinnamon and nutmeg, and broiled in a toaster oven or broiler.
- A smoothie made of 1 cup blueberries or other fruit, 1 banana (try freezing it first), rice or soy milk, and 1 cup plain organic yogurt.
- Whole grain toast with nut or seed butter.
- Yogurt Nut Butter Blend: 3 tablespoons almond butter (or other nut or seed butter) stirred into a cup of organic plain yogurt.
- Cottage Cheese Nut Butter Blend: 2 tablespoons tahini (or other nut or seed butter) stirred into 1 cup organic cottage cheese.
- Scrambled Eggs or Tofu: scramble 2 organic eggs or 1 cup tofu with soy or other milk, ¼ cup organic cottage cheese or 1 ounce hard cheese, ginger, and turmeric.
- Old Fashioned Muesli (2 servings): Mix 1 cup uncooked quick 1-minute oats, ¼ cup wheat germ, ¾ cup soy or rice milk, ¼ cup orange juice, ¼ cup chopped nuts. Optional: add ¼ cup raisins. Cover and let sit overnight or 8 hours in refrigerator. Add milk if needed before eating.
- Nutritious shakes and smoothies made from fermented soy, vegetable, nut or whey powders, organic yogurt, soy or rice milk, wheat germ, and fresh or frozen fruits including blueberries, strawberries, peaches, and bananas.
- Fruit salads with grapefruit, strawberries, blueberries, raspberries, apples, granola, cinnamon, and organic yogurt.
- 1 or 2 organic eggs seasoned with ginger and turmeric or other spices.
- 1 cup blueberries or seasonal fruit
- Vegetable and unsweetened fruit juices of carrots, spinach, kale, beets, tomatoes, grapefruit, apples, or a combination of a variety of fruits and vegetables. (Avoid sugars and artificial sweeteners.)

Suggestions to include in Lunches. Many of these are described in the Chapter 3 menus:

- Spinach salad (makes 2 portions): 4 cups spinach; 1 avocado; 1 cup cooked beans, rice, fish, or tempeh; 2 tablespoons sesame seeds; 2 tablespoons flaxseed oil or olive oil; turmeric; ginger; favorite spices; and lemon juice.
- Oven-roasted vegetables: Mix vegetables (squash, peppers, etc.) with 2 tablespoons olive oil. Add ginger, turmeric and other herbs and roast as you would for oven roasting vegetables. Add 1 tablespoon sesame seeds and ½ to ¾ cup tempeh or fish (albacore, wild salmon, etc.).
- Stir-Fry (2 portions) about 2 cups vegetables (broccoli, cauliflower, etc.) with 2 tablespoons olive oil and 1 cup tofu. Mix in 1 cup chickpeas or beans or 1 cup cooked wild or brown rice. Add 1 small can water chestnuts, a sprinkle of tamari sauce, turmeric, ginger, and dash of cayenne pepper. (Stir-fries can include nuts, seeds, tempeh, and salmon or other fish.)
- Fresh steamed vegetables (2 portions): Steam about 2 cups of vegetables (broccoli, cauliflower, etc.). Mix in 1 cup tempeh, fish (albacore, wild salmon, etc.), or tofu. Add 2 cups cooked rice noodles, tamari sauce, turmeric, ginger, spices, and 1 tablespoon olive oil, flaxseed oil, or nut butter.
- Stuffed Pita bread (or bread): Combine ½ to ¾ cup humus or mashed tofu, tempeh, or fish (albacore, wild salmon) with 2 to 3 tablespoons of plain yogurt, ginger, turmeric, and a generous amount of spinach and tomatoes. Stuff into pita bread.
- Open-faced tuna or salmon melt: Mix ½ cup or small can of tuna or salmon with 1-2 tablespoons organic plain yogurt, 2 tablespoons organic cottage cheese, dill weed, ginger, and turmeric. Load onto 2 slices of toast and broil in toaster oven or broiler for 4 to 5 min. This can also be made into a sandwich. Hard-boiled egg, tempeh, or tofu may be substituted for fish. You may also substitute 1 ounce hard cheese for cottage cheese.
- Grilled vegetables with almonds, wild rice, and tempeh, tuna, or salmon.
- Salads with your choice of spinach, lettuce, broccoli, cauliflower, zucchini, bell pepper, other veggies, sprouts, tofu or tempeh, beans, lentils, chickpeas, rice, organic cottage cheese, plain yogurt, salmon, tuna or other fish, avocado, nuts, seeds, olives, artichoke hearts, potatoes, olive oil, lemon juice, flaxseed oil, ginger, turmeric, and Italian spices.

• Vegetable bean soups using beans, lentils, or chickpeas and a variety of vegetables.
• Beans, lentils, or chickpeas and wild or brown rice or quinoa.
• Vegetable and unsweetened fruit juices of carrots, spinach, kale, beets, tomatoes, grapefruit, apples, or a combination of a variety of fruits and vegetables.

Suggestions for Snacks. Many of these are described in the Chapter 3 menus:

• 1 piece or 1 cup of fruit.
• Vegetable juice.
• Unsweetened fruit juice. (Avoid sugars or artificial sweeteners.)
• Celery, carrots, radishes, and olives.
• One 6 ounce container organic yogurt or 1 ounce of organic cheese.
• A small handful of almonds or pumpkin seeds.
• 1 celery stalk stuffed with nut butter.

At night, if you are feeling weak or need extra energy, you can have a glass of rice or soy milk or vegetable juice, a cup of clear soup, a cup of tea with milk in it, an organic yogurt cup, a piece of fruit, or warm milk/soymilk with cinnamon and nutmeg.

Have you been eating in an unrestricted manner for a long time? If so, it may be difficult for you to stop eating once you begin even though you have had enough. Try making meals of soups, juices, and healthy shakes to help you to feel full. Then take a ten minute break from eating before you have overeaten. After ten minutes you may find you don't need to begin eating again until your next meal.

Continue to Exercise

Review Section *2.5. A TEN-MINUTE MAXIMIZED WORKOUT* and the exercises presented for the 10 days of the *Dream Diet* in Chapter 3. Also look over the additional exercises presented in Appendix 3. In addition, you can add any type of vigorous exercise to your daily life. As the years pass by, your healthy life may depend on whether you decide to incorporate daily exercise into your schedule.

* * * * * * * * * * * * * * * * * * *

SECOND MALE MUSING ON EXERCISE

If you are able to perform the exercises shown in this book for ten days, that is a praiseworthy accomplishment! Can you continue for another ten days? Ten more? Great! Whoops, you missed a few days there. Oh, no. It's getting kinda old. It isn't fun. It's too much like work. You ask yourself: Do I really want to follow this same exercise routine for the rest of my life?

Well, if you stop, then the benefits you gained with a strong start will be lost within a short time period. You'll be back where you started, except you will be stronger in the discouragement department.

Why did Debra make the suggested exercises so quick and easy? It's simple – to maximize the chance that you will actually **do** them despite your busy schedule and dislike of exercise. Some readers will be happy to follow this basic routine indefinitely. While Debra would like you to exercise your major muscle groups indefinitely through some type of resistance training, this particular workout-routine may just be a starting point for you. For all I know, in a few years you'll be a distance runner or a mountain climber, or maybe a very happy cyclist or cross country skier.

Here are some ideas for enhancing and diversifying your exercise:

1. When using weights or machines, try listening to news or music or exercising with a friend to make the experience more fun.

2. If possible, exercise outdoors part of the time. I truly enjoy a run on a beautiful trail!

3. Find athletic games and activities you like and have fun with your friends and family. I'm not talking about bowling or golf, but something that really gets your pulse going like tennis, basketball, swimming, cross-country skiing, aggressive hiking, and bicycle riding.

4. Pursue the widest variety of activities that your abilities, your schedule, and the weather allow. It will be fun and interesting, and the cross training will give you balanced muscle development and help avoid stress-related injuries to particular joints and muscles.

5. Set challenging but achievable goals for yourself and then celebrate your accomplishments. See if you can lift a little heavier weight or do more repetitions, run a little further and faster, make 100 free throws in a row, or

hike or ski a little further. Maybe for once beat your smug neighbor at tennis. The focus can be on growth and accomplishment, not doing an exercise chore.

6. Even on a busy day do a short, basic, weight workout. What is really important is to do **something**, even if only for minutes.

7. Finally, don't hide from your reflection in the mirror. I've heard it said that by the time we can afford a bathroom with floor to ceiling mirrors, we don't want to look. It doesn't have to be that way! Go ahead and admire the progress you are making. Decide how good you want to look and go for it.

Just as with eating choices, you need to sample and discover the exercise methods that are most effective and enjoyable for you, and then make them an integral part of your daily life. As you become stronger, you will find more challenging activities becoming feasible. Let success beget more success. Your new active life will be more fun than you ever dreamed possible!

* * * * * * * * * * * * * * * * * * * *

Get Enough Sleep

Review Section 2.6. SLEEP. Sleep is not a waste of time! It is hugely beneficial to our health and mental outlook. When well-slept your awake time will be happier and more productive, and you will think more clearly. Getting adequate sleep will also help you lose weight. As mentioned in Section 2.6, there is a link between lack of sleep and excess body weight. In addition, during sleep important biochemical processes occur that are critical to the healthy functioning of our bodies, including important immune functions that help fight disease.

You can also be a good model for your children since sleepless nights are linked to obesity in children. Researchers have found that getting a good night's sleep reduces a child's chances of being obese, and that getting at least 9 hours and 45 minutes of sleep per night significantly lowered the chances of obesity in later life. It was shown that every additional hour of sleep per night a child gets at the age of 8 or 9 reduces the risk of obesity at the age of 11 or 12 by 40%. A study showed that 6th graders who slept for a shorter duration than other 6th graders were more likely to be overweight. The study also showed that children who slept for a shorter duration in the 3rd grade were more likely to be overweight later in the 6th grade, which was independent of whether the child was overweight in the 3rd grade. These researchers concluded that one preventive approach to obesity may be to ensure adequate sleep in childhood.[117]

Being overweight also makes a person more likely to snore, which is often a problem for people who are both overweight and sleep-deprived. A growing number of studies have linked snoring to heart disease and stroke. Both obesity and fatigue exacerbate snoring. Snoring indicates that airflow is restricted. According to researchers, when people are snoring they are struggling so hard to breathe that they are putting stress on their hearts.[118] A further obesity-related problem is sleep apnea.[119] Some researchers believe that people who do not correct their snoring will eventually develop sleep apnea as they age, especially if they gain weight.[120] Obstructive sleep apnea occurs when loud snoring is frequently interrupted by episodes of stopped breathing. The severity of the disorder varies from having the airway close or collapse for seconds to minutes, to a partial closing of the airway, in which the sleeper gets less than a full breath. During as much as half of their sleep time, people with sleep apnea can have lower oxygen concentrations in their blood. This lack of oxygen causes the heart to pump harder to circulate blood faster and over time can lead to irregular heartbeats or high blood pressure.[121] A person with sleep apnea stops breathing for up to 60 seconds or even longer, which can occur hundreds of times per night. Yikes!

The primary dangers connected with sleep apnea are its association with high blood pressure or hypertension,[122] heart problems, fluctuations in blood pressure and heart rate, cardiovascular problems, fragmented sleep, increased sympathetic (nervous system) activity, cortical (brain) arousal, cognitive and behavioral problems,[123] strokes, and the drowsiness that can cause accidents. Sleep apnea is also believed to be linked with both glucose intolerance and impaired insulin function, which are associated with the onset of Type II

---

[117] Pediatrics v.120, No.5, p.1020-1029, November 2007

[118] Science News v.157, No.11, p.172, 3/11/00; Robert Clark of Regional Sleep Disorders Center at Columbus Community Hosp.

[119] The Promise of Sleep, William C. Dement, M.D., Ph.D., Delacorte Press 1999 p.168,178,177,174,181

[120] Regina Walker of Loyola University Medical Center, Science News v.157, No.11, p.172, 3/11/00

[121] Science News v.157, No.11, p.172, 3/11/00

[122] Hypertension. v.42, p.1067, 11/10/03

[123] JAMA v.291, p2013, 4/28/04

diabetes.[124]   There are several treatments for sleep apnea including *weight loss*, continuous positive airway pressure machines, surgery, and medications.[125]   The one non-invasive, potentially curative treatment is *weight loss*.

In general, while individuals can vary, it is accepted that adults need approximately 7 to 8 hours of sleep in a 24-hour period, children and teenagers require more sleep, and older adults may require slightly less. Don't sabotage your future by carrying excess weight, not exercising, and not getting adequate and healthy sleep. Also, don't eat extra food to obtain the energy you should be getting from sleep. Get quality sleep.

Generally Accepted Tips on Improving Sleep and Getting to Sleep:

(1) Do not eat within 3 or 4 hours of bedtime (not a problem for *The 3:00 PM Secret* lifestyle!);

(2) Avoid caffeine in the afternoon and evening;

(3) Maintain a regular bedtime schedule;

(4) Relax before going to bed (reading);

(5) Keep your bedroom quiet throughout the night or use white noise;

(6) Maintain your room at a comfortable temperature;

(7) Keep the bedroom dark and use dim nightlights to avoid turning on bright lights during your sleep hours;

(8) Exercise regularly;

(9) Stop your activities, especially turn off the television, 9 hours before you have to get up, and use the last hour to get ready for bed and for the next day.

A top priority should be soundly sleeping 7 to 8 hours every night.

---

[124] Science News v.166, No.13, p.195, 9/25/04

[125] Crit Rev Oral Biol Med, v.15, No.3, p.137, 2004; American Journal of Respiratory and Critical Care Medicine v.159, No.6, p.1884, June 1999; Chest, v.109, p.1346, 1996, American College of Chest Physicians; Promise of Sleep Delacorte Press 1999 p.181,186-90

PART III

Appendix 1

NOTES ON NUTRITION
AND ORGANIC FOODS

Vegetables, Fruits, and Plant-Based Foods

The U.S. Departments of Agriculture and Health and Human Services suggest eating 3 to 5 servings of *vegetables* and 2 to 4 servings of *fruits* every day.[126] Hundreds of research studies have demonstrated the beneficial health effects of eating fruits and vegetables and that a diet rich in fruits, vegetables, and plant-based foods lowers the risk of developing cancer and other diseases. You cannot eat too many vegetables and fruits!

Fats

Fats are the primary components of our brains, nervous system, cell membranes, eyes, adrenal glands, and male testes. Fats are involved in vital functions in our bodies including the synthesis of hormones and maintenance of nerves, skin, cell membranes, nervous system, brain, and mucous membranes. They are also involved in healthy functioning of the immune, reproductive, cardiovascular, endocrine, digestive, and central nervous systems. Fats facilitate oxygen transportation, stabilize blood sugar, and are involved in absorption of calcium and the fat-soluble vitamins (A, D, E, and K). They also influence blood pressure and affect inflammation, allergies, and pain sensitivity. Fats are an important part of a healthy diet, and avoiding all types of fats is not the way to slim down.

Most people consume a lot more omega-6 than omega-3, so it is important to emphasize omega-3 rich foods such as fish and flaxseed oil or take supplements. The essential *omega-3* fatty acids are found in flaxseed oil; fish oil; cold-water and fatty fish including salmon, tuna, cod, halibut, anchovy and shrimp; flaxseeds; pumpkin seeds; walnuts; canola oil; dark green leafy vegetables; sea vegetables; soybeans; wheat germ; and sprouts. Flaxseed oil and fish are the richest sources. The essential *omega-6* fatty acids are found in evening primrose oil, raw nuts and seeds, legumes, leafy green vegetables, meats, grains, borage oil, black currant seed oil, gooseberry oils, and grapeseed oil. Vegetable oils, such as corn, safflower, sunflower, soybean, cottonseed, and sesame also contain omega-6 fatty acids, although these oils are generally processed and hydrogenated and should be avoided as they contain dangerous transfats. The *omega-9* fatty acids also called *monounsaturated fatty acids*, are not essential but have tremendous health benefits. Good sources of monounsaturated fats include olive oil, avocados, and nuts such as almonds, pistachios, pecans, cashews, hazelnuts, macadamia nuts, and peanuts.

Protein

Proteins are essential for the functioning of our bodies and are generally involved in production, growth, repair and maintenance of cells, tissues, hormones, enzymes, muscles, skin, organs, blood, blood cells, connective tissue, bones, neurotransmitters, the immune system, antibodies, hair, nails, and antioxidants, as well as wound healing, brain function, and stabilizing blood sugar. More specifically, proteins are involved in building muscle tissue, increasing metabolism, growth and repair of cells and tissues, hormone production, enzyme production, neurotransmitter production, function of the immune system, antibody production, fluid balance, wound healing, antioxidant activity, brain function, stabilizing of blood sugar, hair and nail growth, growth-hormone production, production of the pancreatic hormone glucagon, and maintenance of muscles, skin, organs, blood, blood cells, connective tissue, bones, and the nervous system.

If you do not eat meat and have a mostly vegetarian diet, make sure you obtain adequate protein. You may also be somewhat deficient in vitamin B12 as well as zinc and should talk to your doctor about taking B12 and zinc supplements along with a good multi-vitamin/mineral supplement.

Sugars and Carbohydrates

Research studies have found that people who eat a diet high in *sugars* and low-fiber *carbohydrates* are more likely to become diabetic than those who eat less refined foods.[127]   The over-consumption of carbohydrates is implicated in the proliferation of adult-onset diabetes, which is a progressive, serious illness with complications such as kidney failure, heart disease, stroke, blindness, nerve damage, circulatory problems, wound healing problems often resulting in amputations, male impotence, and other debilitating health problems.   Adult-onset diabetes can develop when the insulin secreted into the bloodstream is insufficient or is unable to effectively balance blood sugar levels and store the blood sugar glucose in the muscles. There is also a connection between chronically high insulin levels in the blood and Alzheimer's disease. In fact, people with Type II diabetes, which is characterized by high levels of insulin circulating in the blood, have an increased risk of Alzheimer's disease. Several studies have shown that people with Type II diabetes have twice the risk of developing the disease as non-diabetics.[128]

Low-fat, low-protein, high-carbohydrate diets used to be popular in the U.S. because they had been thought to be helpful in reducing heart disease and some cancers. It turns out that plant-based diets that are not low-fat, but rich in unsaturated fatty acids and include nuts, seeds, fish, olive oil, and oils from grains, nuts, seeds, and fish, do not increase but actually reduce the risk of heart disease. In addition, a study found that colon cancer patients were twice as likely as other people to regularly eat carbohydrate-rich high-glycemic index foods, which release sugar rapidly and put a high insulin demand on the body.[129] Sugar is probably one of the most dangerous natural foods we eat in large quantities. See the Appendix 1 of *The 3:00 PM Secret: Live Slim and Strong Live Your Dreams* for more information on the effects of sugar in the diet.

Simple carbohydrates, or *sugars,* consist of one or two sugar molecules and include table sugar, brown sugar, honey, corn syrup, glucose (dextrose), sucrose, barley malt, maltodextrin, sucrose, fructose in fruits, and lactose in milk

---

[127] JAMA v.277, No.6, p.472, 1997

[128] Science v.301, No.5629, p.40, 7/4/03

[129] Science News v.157, No.19, p.298, 5/6/00

and milk products. Simple sugars are absorbed quickly into the bloodstream and raise blood sugar rapidly. Complex carbohydrates are made up of chains of simple sugars and are found in a variety of foods such as grains, vegetables, beans, legumes, and starches. *Starches* are a family of carbohydrates that consist of linked glucose molecules. Complex carbohydrates generally absorb more slowly providing a steadier blood sugar rise. Some complex carbohydrates found in foods such as carrots, potatoes, white rice, and corn, however, have a high glycemic index and break down quickly causing a rapid increase in blood sugar. The *glycemic index* measures how fast carbohydrates are absorbed into the bloodstream and raise the blood sugar level. Processed complex carbohydrates have been refined to the point that they behave more like simple carbohydrates and break down quickly causing a rapid increase in blood sugar levels. Processed carbohydrates include pasta, white flour, white rice, breads, muffins, bagels, pastries, and most commercial cereals.

The carbohydrates we eat should be primarily complex and have a low glycemic index. A glycemic index above 70 percent represents foods that absorb quickly and raise the blood sugar rapidly; a glycemic index under 40 percent represents foods that absorb slowly and raise the blood sugar more slowly; and a glycemic index between 40 and 70 represent foods that absorb and raise blood sugar moderately. Following are examples of carbohydrate-containing foods having high, moderate, and low glycemic indexes:[130]

Carbohydrate-rich foods with high glycemic index (70 to 100):

Refined breakfast cereals, sugar, honey, white bread, most crackers, graham crackers, white rice, rolled oats, oat bran, cookies, cakes, pastries, whole-wheat bread, corn chips, white bagels, croissants, pretzels, carrots, baked potatoes, cooked potatoes, jams, bananas, pineapples, and raisins.

Carbohydrate-rich foods with moderate glycemic index (40 to 70):

Macaroni, spaghetti, pasta, rye, bulgur, wheat kernels, barley, whole-grain pumpernickel, wheat grain, barley grain, cracked wheat, cracked wheat bread, whole grain breakfast cereals, wild rice, brown rice, peas, navy beans,

---

130
　Science News v.157, No.15, p. 236, 4/8/00; American Journal of Clinical Nutrition v.76, No.1, p.5-56, 2002

lima beans, pinto beans, green beans, corn, popcorn, yams, grapes, oranges, apricots, kiwi, and strawberries.

Carbohydrate-containing foods with low glycemic index (0 to 40):

Peanuts, nuts, soybeans, green vegetables, kidney beans, lentils, chickpeas (garbanzos), tomatoes, tomato soup, milk, plain yogurt, grapefruit, cherries, apples, pears, plums, and peaches.

Eating proteins, fats, and low-glycemic index foods along with high-glycemic index foods can help the high-glycemic index foods absorb more slowly as they mix together. Plant-based foods that are very low in sugar and do not raise blood sugar rapidly include olives, olive oil, lettuce, cucumbers, radishes, peppers, celery, alfalfa sprouts, asparagus, green beans, cabbage, cauliflower, eggplant, scallions, onions, leeks, spinach, squash, pumpkin, snow peas, broccoli, kale, avocados, tomatoes, water chestnuts, artichoke hearts, Brussels sprouts, and bean sprouts. Plant-based foods that have a low glycemic index are also generally high in fiber, which provides a sense of fullness and is beneficial for elimination.

Thoughts on Organic Foods

When you shop, choose organic, no pesticide, no hormone foods. Also, most processed and packaged foods are full of sugars, unhealthy fats, and a myriad of fillers and ingredients our bodies were not designed to consume or use, so it is best to avoid them. I realize that sometimes more nutritious foods cost more, but if you buy smaller amounts of high quality and nutritious foods that may cost a bit more, the total dollars spent on food will be about the same. Besides, by not filling your shopping cart with unneeded junk foods, you are saving money. There is sufficient evidence that the hormones and pesticides in non-organic animal and plant foods are linked with cancer that it is worth avoiding them.

I would like to highlight the benefits of choosing ***organic foods*** over non-organic foods, and cite a few reasons why it is worth the extra dollars to buy organic. Organic versions of dairy, meat, and produce are available in many supermarkets and health food stores and will help you avoid consuming hormones and pesticides.

Researchers have learned that women with elevated levels of pesticides in their breast tissue have a greater breast cancer risk.[131] A study of workers in the pesticide field found an increase in a number of cancers.[132] Researchers speculate that food contamination by additives and carcinogenic contaminants such as pesticides, nitrates, dioxins and other organochlorines contributed to the increase in the incidence of cancers during the past sixty years. Other contributors include viruses, bacteria, parasites, radioactivity, UV, pulsed electromagnetic fields, polycyclic aromatic hydrocarbons, smoke, formaldehyde, and volatile organic compounds such as benzene and 1,3 butadiene.[133] It seems we are poisoning ourselves through our food and environment. Some researchers believe that fat tissue may act as a reservoir for pesticides and PCBs, which are both associated with an increased risk of cancer in the breast and prostate.[134] Avoiding pesticides, environmental chemicals, and excess body fat by eating uncontaminated nutritious foods and eating lightly can only benefit us.

In the United States cows are injected with the bovine growth hormone, rBGH, which causes an insulin-like growth factor (IGF-1) to be released into the body of the cow. Cows injected with rBGH have been found to have unusually high levels of IGF-1 in their fat and milk. IGF-1 does not break down during pasteurization and digestion and is absorbed from the gastrointestinal tract into the body. IGF-1 promotes breast cancer, prostate cancer, and colon cancer. Studies have suggested excess IGF-1 levels in rBGH milk is a risk factor for breast and colon cancers[135] and have shown a positive correlation between circulating IGF-1 concentration in the blood and risk of breast cancer among premenopausal women.[136] The role of IGF-1 in cancer is supported by epidemiologic studies, which have found that high levels of circulating IGF-1 are

---

[131] http://www.mayoclinic.com/health/breast-cancer-prevention/WO00091

[132] Occupational and Environmental Medicine v.66, No.1, p.7-15 Jan 2009

[133] Biomed Pharmacother v.61, No.10, p.640-58, Dec. 2007; Epub 2007 Nov 20.

[134] Biomedicine and Pharmacotherapy v.61, No.10, p.665-78, Dec. 2007

[135] Journal of the National Cancer Institute v.93, No.3, p.238, 2/7/01

[136] The Lancet v.351, Issue 9113, p.1393, 5/9/98

associated with increased risk of several common cancers, including those of the prostate, breast, colorectum, and lung.[137] There is ongoing research in this area.

I believe spending a few extra dollars on organic foods is well worth it. While occasionally eating small amounts of the harmful substances contained in most processed and non-organic foods is unlikely to have a significant negative effect on one's health, the eventual accumulation of harmful substances put into one's body day after day adds up and can have substantial destructive consequences.

---

[137] Journal of the National Cancer Institute v.92, No.18, p.1472, 9/20/00

Appendix 2

BODY MASS INDEX (BMI)

A transition is underway in the United States to identify and classify overweight and obese adults using body mass index, or BMI. As BMI value increases, the risk for some diseases increases. BMI is calculated using weight and height. To obtain your BMI you can use the chart below. If your height or weight is not listed, or you want to compute your exact BMI value, multiply your weight (in pounds) by 703 and then divide it by your height (in inches) squared, or:

$$\text{BMI} = [(\text{Your weight in pounds})(703)] \div [(\text{Your height in inches})^2]$$
$$= [(\text{Your weight in pounds})(703)] \div [(\text{Your height in inches})(\text{Your height in inches})]$$

		19	**20**	**21**	**22**	**23**	**24**	**25**	**26**	**27**	**28**	**29**	**30**	**35**	**40**
		W E I G H T						**(p o u n d s)**							
	4'10"	91	96	100	105	110	115	119	124	129	134	138	143	167	191
	4'11"	94	99	104	109	114	119	124	128	133	138	143	148	173	198
	5'0"	97	102	107	112	118	123	128	133	138	143	148	153	179	204
H	5'1"	100	106	111	116	122	127	132	137	143	148	153	158	185	211
	5'2"	104	109	115	120	126	131	136	142	147	153	158	164	191	218
E	5'3"	107	113	118	124	130	135	141	146	152	158	163	169	197	225
	5'4"	110	116	122	128	134	140	145	151	157	163	169	174	204	232
I	5'5"	114	120	126	132	138	144	150	156	162	168	174	180	210	240
	5'6"	118	124	130	136	142	148	155	161	167	173	179	186	216	247
G	5'7"	121	127	134	140	146	153	159	166	172	178	185	191	223	255
	5'8"	125	131	138	144	151	158	164	171	177	184	190	197	230	262
H	5'9"	128	135	142	149	155	162	169	176	182	189	196	203	236	270
	5'10"	132	139	146	153	160	167	174	181	188	195	202	207	243	278
T	5'11"	136	143	150	157	165	172	179	186	193	200	208	215	250	286
	6'0"	140	147	154	162	169	177	184	191	199	206	213	221	258	294
	6'1"	144	151	159	166	174	182	189	197	204	212	219	227	265	302
	6'2"	148	155	163	171	179	186	194	202	210	218	225	233	272	311
	6'3"	152	160	168	176	184	192	200	208	216	224	232	240	279	319
	6'4"	156	164	172	180	189	197	205	213	221	230	238	246	287	328
								O V E R W E I G H T					**O B E S E**		

Title: B O D Y   M A S S   I N D E X   (B M I)

http://www.consumer.gov/weightloss/bmi.htm

Note that two people can have the same BMI, but a different percent body fat. For example, a muscular athlete with a low percent body fat may have the same BMI as a person with a higher percent body fat. Similarly, for the same BMI value, women are more likely to have a higher percent body fat than men. While BMI can be valuable for assessing obesity and disease risk, it should be used in conjunction with other risk factors, such as the measure of waist circumference.

* * * * * * * * * * * * * * * * * * *

MALE MUSING ON SIZE CREEP

Clothing manufacturers invented "size creep" so customers feel better about growing larger. Saying "I'm still a size 6" feels good, but probably is not true. As size creep crept in, there was mounting evidence that carrying around even 10 extra pounds also meant higher risks of cancer, diabetes, heart disease, and Alzheimer's disease. Why carry that risk around all day? Fat cells store and secrete chemicals you just don't want in your body! Your health and longevity increase significantly by staying the course in weight control until your BMI is not merely at the upper end of "normal", but closer to the low end of the scale.

You already know the greatest danger in dieting. It's not that you won't lose weight but rather that you will gain it back when the diet is over. Just as the best defense is a good offense, the best way to keep from regaining weight is to maintain the lifestyle and continue to shed excess weight until it's gone. Never scrimp on nutrition for your internal organs, but there's no payoff for nurturing excess fat cells. If you do increase your body mass, let it be in the muscle department! After achieving your initial weight loss goals, consider adjusting the bar downward and not settling for the "normal" quasi-fat physique. The reward for a truly lean and fit body is more than just looking great. It is a better chance for a long and healthy life pursuing your dreams!

* * * * * * * * * * * * * * * * * * *

Appendix 3
EXTRA EXERCISES
Remember to keep breathing and when possible exhale as you lift weights.

Biceps--HAMMER CURL (Repeat 40 times)

<u>Start/Finish</u> position: Stand with feet shoulder-width apart, abdominal muscles tightened, and knees unlocked. Hold dumbbells down close to your sides with palms facing inward.

Keeping your upper arm stationary with elbows near waist and palms facing inward, bend right elbow and raise right dumbbell up to your right shoulder in an arc-motion to the <u>Midpoint</u> position. Pause briefly. Lower right dumbbell back down in an arc-motion to <u>Start/Finish</u> position.

Repeat with left dumbbell.

HAMMER CURL
<u>Start/Finish</u> <u>Midpoint</u>

OVERHEAD PRESS
<u>Start/Finish</u> <u>Midpoint</u>

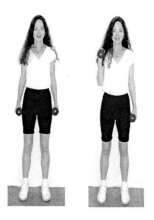
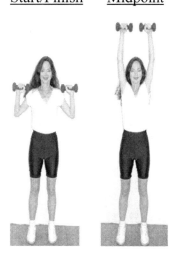

Shoulders--OVERHEAD PRESS (Repeat 40 times)

<u>Start/Finish</u> position: Stand with feet shoulder-width apart, abdominal muscles tightened, and knees unlocked. Hold dumbbells just above shoulders with wrists facing forward and elbows lowered.

Press dumbbells straight up over shoulders keeping wrists facing forward to <u>Midpoint</u> position and continue to press. Pause briefly. Lower dumbbells down to <u>Start/Finish</u> position.

Back--UPRIGHT ROW (*Repeat 40 times*)

<u>Start/Finish</u> position: Stand with feet shoulder-width apart, abdominal muscles tightened, and knees unlocked. Hold dumbbells down in front of legs with palms facing back and the inside ends of the dumbbells touching each other.

Raise dumbbells straight up along the front of your body to your chest keeping your elbows pointing out to the sides, palms facing back, and the inside ends of dumbbells still touching each other to the <u>Midpoint</u> position. Pause briefly. Lower dumbbells back down to <u>Start/Finish</u> position.

UPRIGHT ROW   *FLYE*

<u>Start/Finish</u>   <u>Midpoint</u>   <u>Start/Finish</u>   <u>Midpoint</u>

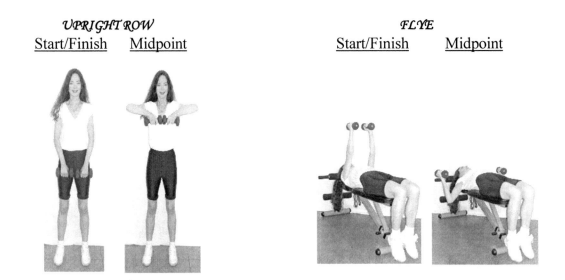

Chest--FLYE (*Repeat 40 times*)

Extra equipment: Weight bench or equivalent.

<u>Start/Finish</u> position: Lie on your back on a bench. Hold dumbbells straight up over your chest with your palms facing each other.

With elbows slightly bent, extend and lower dumbbells out to sides in arc-movements until they are just above chest level (out from your shoulders) at <u>Midpoint</u> position. Pause briefly. While keeping elbows slightly bent but arms extended, raise dumbbells up in arc-movements toward top and center to <u>Start/Finish</u> position.

Triceps--EXTENSIONS (Repeat 40 times)

Start/Finish position: Stand with knees slightly bent (hips forward) and feet about shoulder-width apart or sit on bench with your back straight. Hold each end of a single dumbbell straight up over head with your wrists facing forward and your palms facing up.

While keeping your biceps close to your head, your upper arms pointing up, and your body straight, bend elbows lowering the dumbbell behind your head in an arc-movement to the Midpoint position. Pause briefly. Raise dumbbell back up in an arc-movement to the Start/Finish position.

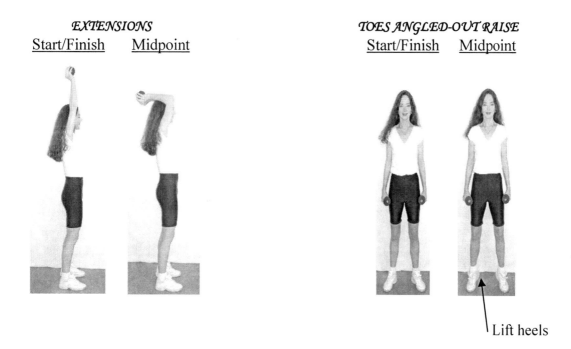

EXTENSIONS   *TOES ANGLED-OUT RAISE*
Start/Finish   Midpoint   Start/Finish   Midpoint

Lift heels

Calves--TOES ANGLED-OUT RAISE (Repeat 40 times)

Start/Finish position: Stand with legs straight and feet shoulder-width apart. Point feet out to sides about half way between forward and sideways and hold a dumbbell in each hand down at your sides with palms facing inward.

While keeping your legs straight, raise up on your toes as far as possible to the Midpoint position.   Lower back down until your heels are touching the floor to the Start/Finish position. Note: Stretch your calf muscles after work out.

Hamstring--CURLS (*Repeat 40 times*)

Extra equipment: Ankle weights.

Start/Finish position: Strap ankle weights onto each ankle and stand up while holding the back of a chair.

Keeping your body and upper legs stationary, bend one knee raising lower leg and foot up in an arc-motion until your knee is at a 90-degree angle and your foot is in the Midpoint position. Pause briefly. Lower foot back down in an arc-motion to Start/Finish position.

Repeat this exercise using the other leg.

<table>
<tr><td colspan="2" align="center">*CURLS*</td><td colspan="2" align="center">*EXTENSION*</td></tr>
<tr><td align="center">Start/Finish</td><td align="center">Midpoint</td><td align="center">Start/Finish</td><td align="center">Midpoint</td></tr>
</table>

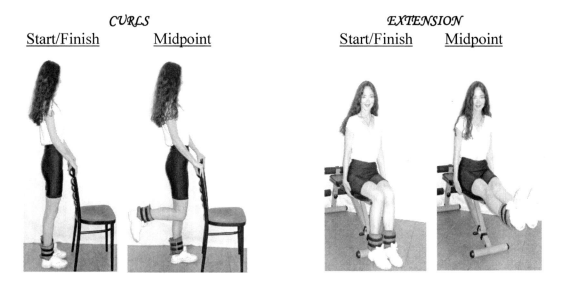

Note: A weight bench with a hamstring curl & extension mechanism may be used.

Quadriceps--EXTENSION (*Repeat 40 times*)

Extra equipment: Ankle weights and a bench or equivalent.

Start/Finish position: Strap ankle weights onto each ankle, sit on a bench with feet down, and hold on to sides of the bench.

Keeping your body and upper legs stationary, extend your lower legs forward in an arc-motion until your knees are straight and your feet are in the Midpoint position. Pause briefly. Lower your feet back down in an arc-motion to Start/Finish position.

FAQs ABOUT THE 3:00 PM SECRET

The following are questions from readers of "*The 3:00 PM Secret: Live Slim and Strong Live Your Dreams*" related to *The 3:00 PM Secret* lifestyle that you may find relevant to your situation:

(1) *I work a swing shift or unusual hours. When do I eat my last meal?*

Eat your last meal 7 to 9 hours before going to bed. The idea of *The 3:00 PM Secret* is to eat your meals early in *"your day"*, so that the calories you eat will be burned for energy while you are active. If, for example, you work a swing shift and arise at 8:00 PM and go to bed at noon, you will want your last meal 7 to 9 hours before you go to bed, or perhaps by 3:00 AM.

To determine when you should have your last meal, count back 7 to 9 hours from your bedtime and eat your last meal before that time. Also, make sure you eat nutritiously and get 7 to 8 hours of sleep. Otherwise, you may be tempted to eat for the energy you should be getting from adequate sleep. If you need a snack during the last 9 hours before bed, try a glass of juice or soymilk, warm milk/soymilk with nutmeg, a piece of fruit, or a small yogurt.

(2) *Does eating about the same amount of food early versus late in the day really make that much difference in whether a person can lose weight?*

Not eating late in the day and at nighttime provides an extraordinary weight-control advantage. Research supports this (see Section 2.3 subsection Why It Works). When you eat during the late afternoon and at night before you become inactive or asleep, much of what you eat is stored in fat cells. Sumo wrestlers learned this trick centuries ago! Doesn't it make sense that if you eat early, you can burn what you eat during the day for energy when you are most active? Alternatively, if you skip breakfast or eat very little food early in the day, you will have less energy, be more lethargic, and burn fewer calories throughout the day as you drag yourself around. Skipping breakfast also makes you more likely to eat an unhealthy, high-calorie, pick-me-up food such as a pastry. Calories eaten early can be burned as you go through your activities of the day and the calories eaten later in the day or evening will be stored as fat.

(3) *What about the cultural tradition of meeting with family over dinner? When would I see my family? How can I give up family time at dinner?*

Is it surprising that our culture is embroiled in an obesity epidemic when people believe they cannot have family time together if it does not involve putting food into their mouths? What is the reality of the dinner ritual? Does it usually involve every member of the family cooking, eating, and cleaning up *together*? No. In fact, it can be a lonely time for the one person tasked with the preparation or cleanup. Instead of a food event, can't a family spend the entire evening together taking a long walk, playing a game or sport, talking about life issues, working on homework and other projects, or reading aloud to each other? Have breakfast as your family mealtime together when you all sit down and discuss the day.

(4) *But my children need to eat dinner. How do I feed them? Also, what if my spouse wants dinner? Sometimes I work fairly late and by the time I get home everyone is hungry.*

If you have slim, active children who need an evening meal and/or a spouse who wants dinner, you can prepare a light, healthy dinner for them and save your portion for the next day's lunch. If you are making a main-dish salad, you can prepare it early and eat your portion early if you are home. Try to prepare your children's dinner as early as possible. Also prepare everyone's lunch for the next day during this time. Satisfy yourself with healthy food early in the day. Slowly move the calorie intake of your entire family to a slightly earlier time when each of you needs the energy. Also, make sure everyone eats a substantial breakfast and lunch. If you often work late, prepare extra food on the weekend that can be eaten during the week. Some dishes can be frozen and then supplemented with fresh ingredients. You can make large main-dish salads, stir fries, etc., two or three times a week that will provide lunches for you and dinners for your children for a few days.

If it is just your children eating dinner, you can sit with them and enjoy a glass of juice or rice or soy milk, or have a yogurt cup or a piece of fruit. If your spouse is eating with your children, you can either sit with them or give your spouse special bonding time with the children and do something for yourself – a bubble bath, call your best friend, or contemplate your life's purpose.

By being slim and active yourself, you will be setting a good example for your children and may be preventing them from ever becoming overweight. Did you know that parental obesity is the greatest predictor of childhood obesity? If you and your spouse both need to lose a few pounds, your children are statistically likely to have weight problems at some point. If your mate sees you slim down, perhaps he or she will want to join you. Try to use evenings to focus on each other and if possible enjoy healthy activities together.

(5) *Going out to dinner is a form of entertainment. What do I do?*

I agree that going out for dinner with friends or a mate can be a fun experience. You can still follow *The 3:00 PM Secret* lifestyle and go out for dinner for special occasions – just not every night! (Trust me – you won't want to.) Are there any other evening activities you can do for entertainment with a friend besides eating? How about joining an astronomy club, playing tennis or golf, running, biking, walking, or cross-country skiing, depending on where you live and the time of year? If you must occasionally have a more culinary experience, how about going out and having **one** very special, expensive glass of wine? When you are not spending all that money on food, you can afford a fancier glass of wine.

The 3:00 PM Secret is such a successful method of weight control, and it feels so good to be light and strong, don't you think it may be worth being a little creative with how you entertain yourself in the evening? *The 3:00 PM Secret* gives you the time to do anything you want with your evenings and frees you from the fix/eat/clean-up dinner tedium. You may discover all sorts of wonderful activities you thought you did not have time for now that you are slim, strong, and feeling unbound!

(6) *Is it OK to go all that time without eating?*

If you are concerned about not eating between 3:00 PM and the next morning, a period of 15 or 16 hours, consider that many people skip breakfast and eat their first meal at noon. These breakfast skippers go without food from sometime between 6:00 PM and 9:00 PM at night until 12:00 PM the next day, which is the same or more hours without food as *The 3:00 PM Secret* suggests – just at the wrong times! In addition, people on a more traditional schedule often eat dinner at 5:30 PM, so there is only about a three-hour difference between not eating after 3:00 PM and not eating after 6:00 PM. If you need it, you can have a glass of vegetable juice, rice or soy milk, or a piece of fruit in the evening.

Appendix 5
NOTES ON AGING

Thoughts from Isabelle... I was surprised to learn that when a test was performed between younger and older typists, the older typists were able to type just as fast as younger typists by reading ahead and anticipating the next key. While the speed of each individual keystroke was a bit slower for the older typist, they compensated by reading ahead.[138] *My research has revealed that although a person may slow down the speed at which she performs certain skills as she ages, she can still accomplish any task – perhaps just a little bit more slowly. In fact, any slowing that may occur as we age is often compensated for by the wisdom and experience we have gained over our lifetimes. I don't know about you, but I think this is great news! I plan to live vigorously through the century mark, and I have every intention of remaining bright, vigorous, and strong. Interestingly, many of the behaviors we apply to keeping our bodies healthy, slim, and fit, will also help us enjoy longer, more vigorous, and happier lives.*

Thanks, Isabelle. The wisdom and experience we gain during life makes us more interesting and valuable as we age. Not only does experience help us when doing projects and tasks, but when it comes to thinking, analyzing, and making decisions, the results regarding aging are quite encouraging. While the speed at which we make decisions may slow somewhat with age, applying wisdom and experience will result in better decisions! Active, stimulated brains do not lose mental abilities with age that cannot be compensated for easily.

Unfortunately some people don't age as well as others. Why? What makes certain people decline with age while others remain strong physically and mentally as the years stream by? A summary of characteristics found in various studies of people who age successfully includes:

Stealing Time: The New Science of Aging, Warshofsky, TV Books 1999 p.17,187,193

(1) higher levels of education and continual intellectual challenge (novelty) all through life;

(2) good nutrition habits;

(3) high levels of exercise and physical activity;

(4) avoiding cardiovascular disease and other life-threatening diseases;

(5) absence of chronic diseases;

(6) avoiding too much stress exposure;

(7) good lung function;

(8) better socioeconomic status and occupation or middle-class lifestyle;

(9) positive emotions;

(10) more adaptive coping skills;

(11) maintaining a feeling of control over one's life;

(12) high intellectual status of spouse;

(13) a flexible approach to life;

(14) being religious; and

(15) being mentally tough.[139]

While lifespan is influenced by our genes, aging is not a preprogrammed process governed directly and completely by our genes. In fact, it is believed that genes do not determine lifespan, but rather genes affect longevity because of their impact on our physiological capacity throughout life.[140] This suggests lifestyle plays a significant role in reducing the effects of aging. This is also consistent with the evidence that lifestyle can significantly increase or decrease our chances of acquiring life-threatening diseases, which has a huge impact on how or whether we age.

Did you know scientists once thought mental decline with age was inevitable? In more recent years they have shown this to be wrong, with some exceptions. Throughout our lives and into old age, we make new connections in our brains from one neuron to another as we learn and put ourselves into stimulating environments. Neurons develop in the adult mammalian brain, including in the hippocampus area of the brain. A number of research studies

---

[139] Stealing Time: The New Science of Aging, Warshofsky, TV Books 1999 p.180,195,205,224-32; p.188-193/Schaie, K.W. Intellectual development in adulthood: The Seattle Longitudinal Study. New York: Cambridge University Press, 1996; Science News v.159,No.2, p324, 5/26/01

[140] Nature v.408, No.6809, p.268, 11/9/00

have shown that neurogenesis occurs in the human brain and that the adult nervous system generates new neurons.[141]

There is more and more evidence our activities can affect new growth in our brains. Studies have demonstrated that physical *exercise* primarily stimulates an increase in *vasculature* and *blood flow* in the brain, whereas *learning* new tasks primarily stimulates *growth of new dendrites* and *synaptic connections* in the brain.[142] Therefore, if we learn new things, we will grow new dendrites and synaptic connections in our brains, and if we exercise, we will increase the vasculature and blood flow in our brains. Which is more important: learning or exercising? Both are enormously important and work in concert.

It has been shown that if we stop using our brains at any age, our dendrites can retract and affect us cognitively. This is similar to a muscle getting smaller if you stop using it. Retracting dendrites can cause a loss in computational power, which is why *continuing to learn and stimulate our brains is so important at any age*. The good news is that dendrites can grow at any age as we use our brains and learn.

In fact, it has been shown that learning alters the structure and function of the brain, and that changes occurring in synapses (the connections between neurons) are associated with different types of learning.[143] Researchers have also shown that intense learning and the acquisition of a great amount of highly abstract information appears to be related to a particular pattern of structural gray matter changes in specific brain areas, showing a significant increase in gray matter.[144]

Why do I cite these studies on brain research (and there are numerous similar studies I could include)? To emphasize that the brain is *dynamic*, and we can improve it and keep it acting young or we can neglect it and let it deteriorate. Just like our muscles, we can strengthen brain connections and computational

---

[141] Science (Adv. online pub.) DOI: 10.1126/science.1136281, 2/15/07; Annual Review of Neuroscience, v.28, p.223, July 2005; Annual Review of Pharmacology and Toxicology, v.44, p.399, February 2004

[142] Beckman News-Summer/Fall 1996 (V. 6/No. 2)/ http://www.beckman.uiuc.edu/outreach/bnfeature96.html; Proceedings of the National Academy of Sciences, v.87, No.14, p.5568-5572, 1990

[143] Curr Opin Neurobiol. v.9, No.2, p.203, Apr.1999 /Science v.289, No.5478, p.399, 7/21/00

[144] The Journal of Neuroscience, v.26,No.23,p.6314, 6/7/06

power with use or let our brains and bodies deteriorate with disuse. The fact that it is possible to keep our brains fully functional well into old age should provide even more motivation to keep our bodies in tip-top shape. Our lifespans can be increased by positive changes we make every day throughout our lives.

So, what will help our bodies stay healthy longer? A number of factors that are known to affect the *aging process* and *lifespan* include: education and continued learning, exercise, stress reduction, antioxidants and vitamins, calorie restriction and being lean, and avoidance of Alzheimer's disease. Making positive changes in lifestyle along with obtaining appropriate medical intervention later in life can notably improve your life expectancy.[145]

Here is some practical advice for reducing the effects of aging:

(1) *Stimulate your brain* through *learning* and exposing yourself to new ideas, new information, challenges, and novelty. Mental activity creates a richer and more redundant array of connections between nerve cells in the brain, and these stronger connections are believed to be better able to resist small insults to the brain that occur over a lifetime. Numerous studies have demonstrated that people with more *education* live longer, postpone the onset of dementia, and reduce the risk of Alzheimer's disease. Even if you did not get a formal education, you can have a great impact on your brain health and cognitive function by engaging in intellectually stimulating and challenging activities now and throughout your life. Reading and other cognitively-challenging activities help you gain better, more resilient neural connections in your brain.[146]

(2) *Exercise*! I believe vigorous daily physical activity is critical to maintaining good health, insuring good brain function, avoiding and recovering from illness or injury, and creating happiness. If you do not engage in daily exercise, it is probably because you either do not think you have time or do not want to find time. That is why I developed the "ten-minute workout". Just do it six days a week. Soon you will recognize the benefits and will want to adopt other more extensive physical activities. Exercise and being lean will help keep you slim, strong, smart, healthy, and beautiful well into your later years!

---

[145] Science v.301, No.5640, p.1679, 9/19/03

[146] Neurology v.69, p.470-476, 7/31/07

(3) *Guard yourself from bad stress.* When we are under stress, stress hormones are released in our bodies. These hormones cause the mobilization of glucose from storage into the bloodstream, an increase in heart rate and blood pressure, and a suspension of various long-term, energy consuming functions, such as digestion, growth, reproduction, tissue repair, and maintenance of the immune system. The chronic production of the stress hormone cortisol that occurs when the body is exposed to continual stress has been linked to heart disease and upper respiratory infections. Prolonged exposure to stress is believed to cause aging in our brains and damage to or loss of neurons in the parts of the brain involved in learning and memory.[147] Discover your dream life, read the Bible, be happy and at peace, and have perspective. Live the life God meant for you to live.

(4) *Eat fruits, vegetables, and plant foods*, with their abundance of vitamins, minerals, phytochemicals, free-radical fighting *antioxidants*, and other beneficial compounds. They will fight off diseases and enhance health, which can help to give you a longer, healthier life. Antioxidants found in fruits, vegetables, plant foods, and supplements can help protect neurons in the brain from damage by free radicals. Fruits and vegetables are also rich in potassium which helps protect and preserve muscle tissue.[148]

(5) *Eat healthy and light.* We learned in Chapter 2 from the 2007 *Report* on cancer that being lean was the panel's first recommendation for avoiding cancer. While I am not advocating "calorie restriction", it is important to understand the health and longevity benefits of eating fewer more nutritious calories. Calorie Restriction is a method that has been shown to extend life in various species of animals, including primates, resulting in the animals actually remaining healthier, more disease free, and physiologically younger at more advanced ages. Calorie-restricted animals show positive physiological changes during their extended life, such as having healthier blood pressures, healthier levels of cholesterol, better levels of HDLs and LDLs, lower triglycerides, and a

---

[147] Curr Opin Neurobiology, v.5, No.2, p.205, Apr.1995

[148] American Journal of Clinical Nutrition v.87, No.3, p.662, March 2008; Science News, v.173, No.13, p.205, 3/29/08

lower risk of heart disease, stroke, cancer, and diabetes.[149] Calorie-restriction involves feeding animals a diet that is **very rich in nutrients** but lower in calories than a normal diet. The benefits of calorie restriction appear to begin at about 10 percent restriction and increase until the restriction approaches 50 percent. Research suggests that having lower body fat can extend a healthy life.[150]

(6) *Avoid Alzheimer's disease*! Alzheimer's disease is physically characterized by abnormal deposits of certain proteins in the brain, specifically beta-amyloid protein plaques and tau protein tangles. It is estimated to affect 25% to 45% of people age 85 and older, although the disease can begin in the 60s. While Alzheimer's disease becomes more common with age, it is not a normal part of aging. Researchers are investigating protective strategies and therapeutic interventions including: education and intellectual stimulation; exercise; not being overweight; omega-3 fatty acids; estrogen therapy used early (currently under investigation); statins (cholesterol-lowering drugs); non-steroidal anti-inflammatory drugs; and antioxidant vitamins, namely E, C, Niacin, and other antioxidants found in fruits, vegetables, and the spice turmeric.[151] Studies suggest intellectual stimulation, education, and physical exercise can reduce Alzheimer's disease risk and push back symptoms. Not surprisingly, television watching is associated with increased incidence![152] Chronically high insulin levels in the blood are also associated with Alzheimer's disease. Likewise, people with Type II diabetes, characterized by high levels of circulating insulin, have twice the risk of developing the disease as non-diabetics.[153] Women who are overweight at age 70 (and in their 70's) have a higher risk of developing Alzheimer's disease and dementia than slimmer women. In fact, for every 1.0 unit increase in BMI at age 70, Alzheimer's disease risk increased by 36%! Besides getting the weight off, researchers are investigating other possible preventatives and treatments which include:

---

[149] Science v.325, No.5937, p.201, 7/10/09; Science News v.176, No.3 p.9, 8/1/09; Science News v.158, No.22 p.341, 11/25/00 and Science News v.151, No.11, p.162, 3/15/97; Stealing Time, Warshofsky, TV Books 1999 p.103-116; also see http://www.walford.com/research.htm

[150] Science v. 304, No. 5678, p.1731, 6/18/04

[151] Omega-3 fatty acids Science News v.166, No.10, p.148, 9/4/04; NSAIDS Science v.302, No.5648, p.1215, 11/14/03; Niacin Science News v.166, No.9, p.142, 8/28/04; Turmeric The Journal of Neuroscience, 11/1/01, v.21, No.21, p.8370; Turmeric BBC NEWS, Wed., 11/21/01

[152] Science v. 309, No. 5736, p 864, 8/5/05

[153] Science v..301, No.5629, p.40, 7/4/03

resveratrol, a compound found in grapes and red wine;[154] a green tea component called epigallocatechin-3-gallate;[155] folates from oranges, legumes, leafy green vegetables, and folic acid supplements;[156] omega-3 fatty acids found in fish[157] and flaxseed oil; and exercising both the body and mind.[158]

Unless you are stricken with a disease in spite of your efforts to ward it off, there is absolutely no reason for your mind and body to significantly deteriorate with age. You may decline somewhat as you push through the century mark, but if you keep your mind and body young and healthy through good nutrition, exercise, and maintaining a healthy low weight, as well as reducing stress, getting enough sleep, and continuing to stimulate your brain through intellectual pursuits, you can stay young mentally and physically well into old age. Find the pursuits that fascinate you and never stop living your dreams!

Knowing that our habits and behaviors can increase our chances of having a longer, healthier life should further motivate us to take care of our minds and bodies now and throughout life.

* * * * * * * * * * * * * * * * * * *

MALE MUSING – DON'T ACT YOUR AGE!

"You need to slow down and act your age. Take it easy on your body." I received this advice on occasion from a parent when I was in early "middle age" and called to share my excitement about accomplishing goals such as a good 10K time or completing a challenging mountain ascent.

Children are often scolded with the rhetorical question "Why don't you act your age?" Who wants to be a baby? Later in life, though, I learned to take these inquiries as compliments. I don't **want** to act my age if that means limiting my activities, scaling back my goals, and turning control of my life over to caregivers. I've always preferred the idea of dying with my boots on, not deteriorating on the

---

154
    Journal of Biological Chemistry November 11, 2005
155
    Journal of Neuroscience Sept. 21, 2005
156
    The Journal of the Alzheimer's Association Inaugural issue 2005
157
    Online issue of the Journal of Neuroscience March 23, 2005
158
    Cell v.120, p.701, 3/11/05

shelf. So, I have rejected the idea of growing old gracefully and prefer to stay young aggressively.

There is a point in life when many people see an unsettling vision of the future. They see all too clearly that they have begun a slow decline, a glide path to the nursing home and idle dependency. They think their best days are over, and the many unachieved goals become receding unattainable mirages. They may have an overwhelming temptation to despair, to sag in spirit, to accept life "as it is", and resign prematurely to the inevitability of old age. Friends and family notice they seem old because they have begun to **think** "old". With help from family they begin to excuse themselves from the more challenging and adventuresome activities they once enjoyed, and reluctantly become better acquainted with sedentary and quiet activities that do not require a strong body or mind. Not surprisingly, it is a self-fulfilling vision of the future. If you think old, you will act old, and before long your body and mind will become old. A return to some level of youthful vigor will appear impossible.

Even if the temptation to despair and give up dreams feels overwhelming, it is important not give in. We all know people who reached the same mid-life crossroads and not only rejected the inevitable, but rebelled against it. They didn't like what they saw down the road and consciously changed the direction of their lives. It took the form of a new career, moving to a new place, going back to school, new recreational or intellectual pursuits, or maybe even a new toupee or hairstyle and a sports car.

Friends and family were surprised by these peculiar, unrealistic, and inappropriate behaviors. Then the "act your age" comments began appearing, possibly from an unconscious envy of a person for achieving what the critic did not or for hoping while the critic felt hopeless. Yet as the years passed, these innovative, forever-young, sparkling people became an inspiration rather than an oddity. Will you be inspired to be one of them? When you're 80 years old, do you want to be ordering more pills for your ailments or purchasing new luggage for your next adventure?

Why are these people inspiring? Isn't it because they have confounded the critics by continuing to live vital and interesting lives that make a difference to themselves and others? The purpose of successful aging is not to see how long you can continue to breathe but to continue to fill your life with enjoyable and useful experiences.

You can begin today fashioning a precious gift to yourself and the people you care about. The gift is a healthy, hearty, and happy you. It is fashioned every day when you keep your body and mind in tune with excellent nutrition, weight control, exercise, sleep, and, most important, purpose. If you stop pursuing worthwhile goals, you won't continue to function mentally or physically.

Why not take secret pleasure in confounding the calendar, the nay-sayers, and even the grim reaper himself? When you reach the crossroads where the main highway is marked "the beginning of the end", consider taking the little unpaved uphill turn that may lead you to many exciting new beginnings. Today you can start making the necessary changes to your lifestyle that will ensure that you'll be fit for the journey.

* * * * * * * * * * * * * * * * * * *

Appendix 6
SHOPPING LIST

The following are minimum amounts estimated for the ten days of the diet for one person. Increase amounts for larger portions or additional people. Note that some lunches give you choices, so look over the menu to decide amounts of tofu, tempeh, fish, beans, or rice to have on hand.

2 cups granola
2 cups oatmeal
7 pieces dense, multigrain bread
3 pita bread
9 cups plain organic yogurt
2 cups organic cottage cheese
6 cups blueberries, strawberries, etc.
1 banana
9 pieces fruit (pear, apple, orange, grapefruit, etc.)
4 cups grapefruit juice or unsweetened fruit juice
4 cups vegetable juice
5 cups vegetables for salad, steam, or stir-fry (broccoli, cauliflower, etc.)
5 to 6 cups spinach
3 to 4 tomatoes
1 avocado
Carrots and celery sticks for snacks
7 tablespoons nut or seed butter (almond butter, toasted tahini, etc.)
Rice milk and/or soy milk for cereal and to drink a cup at night
2 organic eggs (or 1 cup tofu) for "scrambled eggs (or tofu)"
1 small can water chestnuts drained
2 cups cooked rice noodles
1 small can of tuna or salmon
3 to 4 cups humus, tofu, tempeh, or fish (albacore, wild salmon)
1 cup tofu
1 cup garbanzo or other beans, or 1 cup wild or brown rice
1 cup beans, rice, fish, or tempeh
10 walnut or pecan halves
2 tablespoons sesame seeds
Olive oil, lemon juice, and Tamari sauce
Spices: Turmeric, ginger, dill weed, cinnamon, and nutmeg
Flaxseed oil or fish oil supplements or flaxseed oil for daily consumption

(Cutout or photocopy)

Chart Your Future
After completing your first 10-Day Dream Diet
<u>*make 12 copies of this page and fill it in each month for a year.*</u>

Today's Date is:_____   My weight is:_____lbs

I. Continue the Dream Diet lifestyle by: Not eating meals 7 to 9 hours before bedtime; eating nutritiously (Chapter 3's Menus, Ten Nutrition Tips in Section 2.4, and What Foods to Focus On and Ideas for Meals in Chapter 5); exercising vigorously at least ten minutes daily; getting 7 to 8 hours of sleep; and discovering and living your dreams. How well are you doing?

_____

_____

_____

II. Reread your answers to the ten Dream Questions. Write down any changes you would make to your answers of Dream Questions 1 through 8.

_____

_____

_____

III. Do you still agree with the 5 dreams you listed in Question 9(A)? Rewrite them, making any changes that reflect your most recent thoughts.

1._____

2._____

3._____

4._____

5._____

IV. Describe your dream body as you did in Dream Question 9(C). How close are you to achieving it, and what do you still need to do?

_____

_____

V. How are you pursuing your dream life (see Question 10(A))?

_____

_____

_____

Other Books by These Authors
~ Available on-line or through bookstores ~
See ***www.GlacierDog.com***

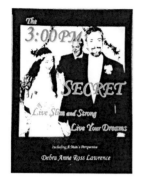

The 3:00 PM SECRET
Live Slim and Strong Live Your Dreams

The foundational book that develops the philosophy and practical steps that will make you slim, strong, and healthy. "The 3:00 PM SECRET is unique because of its motivation and its simple and innovative approach to eating. Living The 3:00 PM SECRET is so easy and such a positive experience, it seems like magic."

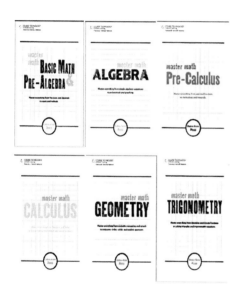

MASTER MATH Books
Basic Math and Pre-Algebra
Algebra
Geometry
Trigonometry
Pre-Calculus
Calculus

These best-selling books, now in second editions, explain principles, definitions, and operations of each subject, provide step-by-step solutions, and present examples and applications. These comprehensive books teach in a way that is easily understood by students of all ages!

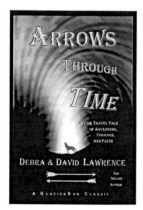

ARROWS THROUGH TIME
A Time Travel Tale of
Adventure, Courage, and Faith

"A must read for anyone fascinated by time travel and its possibilities. An intriguing, insightful, and inspiring tale of faith, fate, and heroism with compelling characters and surprising twists. This fun, fast-moving adventure will take you on an unforgettable journey."

LaVergne, TN USA
07 January 2010

169210LV00005B/2/P